D0994092

Breast is Best

Penny and Andrew Stanway are London-trained doctors who were married in 1969. They have three young children, all of whom were breastfed.

Penny Stanway has spent time in general practice and in research. During her appointment as senior medical officer to a large area health authority and while breastfeeding her first child she found that there was a need for an up-to-date book about breastfeeding. She is particularly interested in the prevention of disease and in child care and has written widely for magazines and journals on these subjects. She has co-authored five books with her husband. Although she has temporarily retired from practising medicine in order to be a full-time mother, she is a member of the Professional Advisory Board of La Leche League International and a member of the Panel of Advisers to the National Childbirth Trust, and she devotes much of her professional energy to the promotion and encouragement of breastfeeding.

Andrew Stanway was a medical registrar at a London teaching hospital until twelve years ago. He now lectures, broadcasts, writes and makes films on medical topics both for the medical and dental professions and for the general public. He has written twelve books including *Taking the Rough with the Smooth*, about dietary fibre, an *Encyclopaedia of Alternative Medicine*, *Overcoming Depression*, *Why Us?* – a guide for infertile couples – and, jointly with his wife, *The Breast Book*, the *Pears Encyclopaedia of Child Health*, *The Baby and Child Book*, and *The Complete Book of Love and Sex*, to be published soon.

Andrew and Penny Stanway are active in promoting breastfeeding worldwide and have many years' experience in counselling mothers with breastfeeding problems.

Also by Penny and Andrew Stanway in Pan Books
The Baby and Child Book
Choices in Childbirth
Also by Andrew Stanway in Pan Books
Taking the Rough with the Smooth

Penny and Andrew Stanway

Breast is Best
a common-sense approach to breastfeeding

Foreword by Dr Hugh Jolly MA MD FRCP DCH

Pan Original
Pan Books London and Sydney

For Susannah, Amy and Ben

First published 1978 by Pan Books Ltd.
Cavaye Place, London SW10 9PG
9 printings
This revised edition published 1983
19 18 17 16
© Penny and Andrew Stanway 1978, 1983
ISBN 0 330 28110 0
Photoset by Parker Typesetting Service, Leicester
Printed and bound in Great Britain by
Collins, Glasgow

Contents

Foreword by Hugh Jolly MA MD FRCP DCH

This book, while written for parents, should convince doctors and nurses as well as the parents themselves that there is a need for another book on breastfeeding. Unfortunately, there is still serious ignorance amongst those whose task it is to advise mothers, with the result that they are bombarded by differing advice as to how to breastfeed successfully. This is not due to changes in fads and fashions but to a lack of training in the physiological processes of lactation which are so well set out in this book.

I started writing this foreword while working in the Middle East. I was appalled to hear young British midwives advising Arab mothers on breastfeeding, describing methods which should have been discarded years ago. The clock has no part to play in breastfeeding and yet these mothers were being told to feed three-hourly or four-hourly. This could have been correct if they had been veterinary surgeons advising farmers about the feeding of calves but, because of the enormous differences in the composition of cows' milk compared with human milk and in the very growth processes of babies and calves, it was totally incorrect for human mothers. I also keep hearing the appalling advice to feed 'ten minutes each side'. Whoever first invented that catchphrase had no knowledge of the physiology of lactation.

Fortunately, all this is explained here in a straightforward and understandable manner. As the authors describe the latest information on the difference between human milk and cows' milk, one is left with the nightmare this must mean for the manufacturers of cows' milk preparations. Their present attempts to modify cows' milk cannot hope to keep up with the advances in our understanding of the composition of human milk. One can only pity them their impossible task as they dismantle and convert their manufacturing plants.

On the other hand, one is left feeling enormous relief for today's mothers who have no need to worry about the problems raised by feeding cows' milk to their babies. In fact, the more that is discovered about breast milk the more incredible it seems that we ever stopped using it.

It is so important for mothers to realise that failure to breastfeed results from a lack of the right sort of help rather than from their genes. There is so much more to breastfeeding than just getting food into the baby, but it is not difficult to achieve if the atmosphere is right. My most enjoyable hospital work in the week is the morning's round in the maternity ward where I sit in turn on each new mother's bed and talk with her and her husband about breastfeeding.

I warmly recommend the Stanways' book to all mothers. They will not only learn the enormous advantages to themselves and their babies from breastfeeding, but will be armoured against the ignorant 'advice' which every breastfeeding mother still has to face.

Preface

'Why a book about breastfeeding? Surely it's the most natural thing in the world . . . you don't need to learn about it.'

This is typical of the response we had when we told doctors and lay people alike that we were writing this book. But if it *is* so natural to breastfeed it would be interesting to know why so many women in the western world simply can't do it.

The answer is that it *is* natural but the ability to do it successfully doesn't necessarily come naturally. To those mothers who find breastfeeding easy, a book such as this may seem a complete waste of time but we hope it will be a help to those who don't.

Of all the phases in a woman's reproductive life, lactation has been the least understood and the most debased. At a time when we know more about female sexuality and reproductive life than ever, there is still appalling ignorance about breastfeeding. Unfortunately, this ignorance spreads right through the medical and nursing professions and so makes it very difficult for today's mothers to know where to turn for good advice. This has been made even more difficult because medical advice itself has changed so often.

What we have aimed to do is to clarify this confusion and in so doing to cut away all the 'mumsy' talk so often associated with breastfeeding advice. This isn't because we're insensitive to the emotional and spiritual bonds that exist between a mother and her child but rather because experience has taught us that today's mother wants facts and straight talking first. For this reason you'll find that there are areas in which we have been very brief: we have made an effort not to fill the book with theories and suppositions, nor to mention the old wives' tales that abound elsewhere!

In order to help the reader learn how to breastfeed successfully and cope with any problems, we've screened the world's literature, drawn evidence from a large number of medical journals and talked to experts with a wealth of experience in three continents. Most important, though, we've listened to mothers.

This is not a 'roses round the door' book to make women feel they ought to breastfeed even if they don't want to. No one has the right to do that. We have, however, presented the evidence in favour of breastfeeding in a way that even the most sceptical or half-hearted person should find acceptable.

Some people consider breastfeeding to be unimportant today because of the practical alternative available, while others think that it is an essential part of good mothering. Both views are, of course, extreme but it's surprising how difficult it is to discuss breastfeeding because the whole subject has become such an emotive one.

If you want to breastfeed – or help somebody else to – read on. Millions of women the world over cope perfectly well . . we in the West have simply lost the knack.

Dr Penny Stanway MB BS LRCP MRCS
Dr Andrew Stanway MB MRCP

1 So you want to breastfeed

'Why on earth should I need a book to teach me how to breastfeed?' we can hear you saying. 'Haven't women fed their babies for millions of years? And how do all the millions of women in developing countries get on? They all breastfeed and they don't learn from books.'

Fashions, instinct and education

The answer is more complex than it seems, as any failed breast-feeding mother knows. We live in a society in which breastfeeding has become unfashionable and at a time when many young mothers go into pregnancy never having seen anyone breastfeeding. Because breastfeeding has fallen from grace in the eyes of modern women (and men), it no longer comes instinctively to many mothers and has to be learnt just like any other skill. In fact, it probably never has been entirely instinctive but, in the past, other women helped and taught the new breastfeeding mother, which ensured that breast-feeding was almost universally successful. Evidence from many parts of the world has shown that, in the past, babies of women who failed to produce enough milk simply died. This alone was an enormous incentive for women to help each other to make a success of breastfeeding – as indeed they nearly all did.

Your baby almost certainly won't need to be taught how to feed – that's a natural instinct – but we're a long way from natural instincts so far as the mother's role is concerned today. Most mothers need help and encouragement if they are to succeed.

Before we go any further, let's get one thing straight. With the right advice and encouragement almost every woman can breast-feed happily and successfully for as long as she and her baby want. In 1975, the USA was said to have the lowest breastfeeding rate in the world! Fewer than one in four babies were being breastfed at one week old and by six months the figure had fallen to one in twenty. However, in 1916, 60 per cent of babies were still being breastfed at one year! In evolutionary terms, 1916 is not very long ago at all. In a campaign some years ago to encourage and support breastfeeding in Minneapolis, 96 per cent of nearly 3,000 women were fully breastfeeding when their babies were two months old, and 84 per cent were still breastfeeding at six months. Over the last five years, following the massive publicity about the benefits of breastfeeding and the endorsement of breastfeeding by both the American Academy of Pediatrics and the World Health Organisation, the breastfeeding rate in the USA as a whole has risen to 60 per cent of newborn babies. Following the widespread encouragement of mothers to breastfeed in the UK between 1975 and 1980, two out of every three newborn babies were put to the breast in 1980 compared with one in two in 1975. Though the fall-off rate at present is very rapid once women are back at home and there is obviously plenty of room for improvement, it's clear that mothers *can* breastfeed if they are motivated to and if they are helped enough.

Many people who seriously question why it is that so many western women fail to breastfeed assume that they cannot do so for perfectly good biological reasons. They assume that because bottle-feeding has been practised for so long, the modern woman has become biologically incapable of producing enough milk.

As recently as the beginning of this century the majority of babies in the western world were fed at the breast, and as far as medical science is aware it would take many generations for such a radical biological change to take place – not a mere eighty years. The final condemnation of this argument comes when these so-called 'genetically incapable' women get help and encouragement and go on to feed their babies successfully. *Women fail to breastfeed because of their environment, not because of their genes.*

A study in France showed that the numbers of babies getting *no* breast milk at all rose from 31 per cent to 51 per cent in a matter of five years and over a period of twenty years in Bristol the number of three-month-olds breastfeeding fell from 74 per cent to 36 per cent. These falls are so large and occurred so quickly that no genetic explanation could possibly be acceptable. It had to be an environmental change – a change in attitude.

Man has been on the face of the earth for about five million years yet he has only reared milk-producing animals for the last 10,000 or so of these years. Only in the last fifty years has the use of cows' milk as a source of infant food become widespread. The unnatural change in diet from breast milk to cows' milk at so crucial a period in our lives is a modern intervention without parallel in the history of mankind. So massive and uncontrolled a change is it that it has led one researcher in the field to call it 'the greatest uncontrolled trial ever to have been done on human beings'. Man has become strangely obsessed with cows' milk and this obsession ought to be seriously questioned. The trouble is that in the West the advertising industry, nutritionists and dieticians have made cows' milk into a food with almost magical properties. Could it be that this overemphasis in adult life on the goodness of cows' milk is closely tied (albeit unconsciously) to the fact that we willingly deprive our babies of the very milk they should be getting – their mother's milk?

Why should all this be worrying to the woman who has decided to breastfeed? Today, if a mother has any problems with breastfeeding, she is immediately handicapped further by a sense of guilt and personal failure. Then, because cows' milk formula feeds are so readily available with little fear of personal failure attached she soon starts her baby on the bottle.

The sad part of all this is that breastfeeding is still considered by most people to be simply a way of getting food into a baby. In reality it is so much more.

The first doubts about bottle-feeding started as new facts about the disadvantages of even the newest 'modified' cows' milk formula came to light. Cows' milk preparations were found to lack vitamin B_6, vitamin E and linoleic acid and to be too high in protein, sodium and phosphorus; to cap it all, it was found that there were many more protective antibodies against disease in breast milk than had ever been thought. The discovery was also made that a baby's gut wall could leak whole protein molecules from cows' milk into the bloodstream and that these 'foreign' proteins could lay the foundation for eczema, asthma and other allergic problems both in infancy and in later life.

Baby milk manufacturers speedily changed their formulae to keep pace with these new discoveries and there was talk about vaccinating herds of specially bred cows to give them immunity against human diseases. But by this time the damage had been done and when mothers demanded that they should be allowed to feed their babies with the best baby food of all, they found that the art of breastfeeding had been all but lost. Mothers had lost confidence in their natural ability and common sense and health professionals (doctors and nurses) had seen few mothers successfully breast-feeding and had been brainwashed by rigid advice on schedules for breastfeeding. Hospitals had forgotten that they existed to do their best for the patients and not to idolise the new god, 'routine', and even the mothers' own mothers were often of little help as they had been among the first to use cows' milk when they fed their children.

So this is where we came in. We have found as parents, health educators and doctors that few mothers can get good and consistent advice about breastfeeding. If they can, it tends to stop as soon as they appear to be managing on their own at home. The trouble is that while the new mother might like the idea of breastfeeding, as soon as any problem – however small – crops up, she is lucky if she can continue, because she will be showered with differing advice from all sides. This is especially upsetting as she will probably feel unable to stand up to any upset or to sort out conflicting advice so soon after childbirth. Once she's put the baby on the bottle, she'll feel depressed and guilty. Indeed, many women experience a deep and lasting sense of failure after doing so.

Why you'll need help
Today's society isn't geared to help its young mothers breastfeed, even when they want to. For a start, it's 'normal' for babies to be bottle-fed and if you breastfeed you'll be 'abnormal'. You've got to be prepared for that. Even the 'token breastfeeder' we describe later will not understand the mother who believes in natural breast-feeding. Though more mothers start to breastfeed their babies now, the vast majority of babies are soon completely or almost completely bottle-fed. Statistics in the UK in 1975 showed that only 14 per cent of 'breastfed' babies received *no* cows' milk – and that was the so-called 'breastfed babies'! Mothers who totally and solely breast-feed their babies are rare. No one could argue that anything like 86 per cent of breastfed babies *need* cows' milk, so a lot of babies must have been given it unnecessarily.

A girl can reach motherhood without ever having seen a baby at the breast. Breastfeeding will rarely have been mentioned at school, even in biology and parentcraft classes. Her friends and relatives will be far more familiar with bottle-feeding, and while not actively discouraging her from breastfeeding, they may make a very good job of persuading the mother-to-be that a bottle-fed baby will be as contented and healthy as a breastfed one.

Perhaps more insidious is the fact that today's young woman is brought up and educated to think of herself mainly as a wage-earner and career woman. When she marries, her income will almost certainly be considered necessary to start a home and it's difficult for her to think of giving this up when a baby comes along. She tends to tell herself that she may go back to work part-time soon after the baby is born, or perhaps just a little later. She may even organise things so that she can keep her job and just take maternity leave. In any event, she's not thinking of herself in relation to her baby but rather of her role in relation to her husband and job.

It's often said that today's mother doesn't breastfeed because she has to go back to work so soon. The fact is that only a small percentage of women actually go back to work while their children are really young (see page 149). What a shame they can't admit to themselves that they will be unlikely to go back in the short term and just relax and look forward to being a mother.

Perhaps partly because there is a world population explosion, western society as a whole doesn't value its children and its mothers like it used to. With the downgrading of motherhood in society's eyes it has become widely accepted that any individual mother can easily be replaced by a substitute mother, be she a child minder, a nanny or mother's help, or an au pair. So not only have we accepted the insidiously marketed concept that breast milk is no longer essential for a baby, but we also seem to be accepting the idea that a mother is no longer essential for her baby.

Perhaps the women's movement in the West will be the saving grace for motherhood and breastfeeding, strange though this may seem! Instead of being looked down on by society, women who choose to have, breastfeed and care for their children themselves will hopefully be encouraged not only to think well of themselves for doing a job which is unique for each child, but to enjoy what they are doing and to recognise its tremendous value.

More mothers are showing an interest in breastfeeding today. Unfortunately, their success rates are poor and most of them put this down to 'not having enough milk'. This is completely wrong, as has been shown in studies all over the world. There are very few women who cannot breastfeed if they want to and if they are given enough help.

At this point some readers will be shaking their heads and saying that there is already a lot of help available to the pregnant and nursing mother. However, a large amount of the advice given by doctors and nurses is frankly unhelpful and often contradictory anyway. Why? Mainly because doctors, nurses and midwives are influenced by society and fashion just like the rest of us. They have also been brainwashed over the last fifty years or so into believing that cows' milk formula really is the equal of breast milk. Two recent studies in England bear this out. In one, 355 women were asked what advice they had had during pregnancy about feeding their babies. Three out of four women had had no positive advice to breastfeed and 5 per cent were actually advised to bottle-feed. The second survey found that 81 per cent of women had received no encouragement whatsoever ante-natally. One large UK study in 1975 reported that feeding was not discussed with a doctor or nurse in the case of one out of three pregnant mothers. A follow-up survey five years later showed that feeding was discussed ante-natally with about five mothers out of six, which reflects the increasing awareness of the importance of infant feeding.

We have found that most doctors pay lip service to breastfeeding but won't go all out to convince mothers that it's the very best thing. A survey of American paediatricians showed that they advised mothers according to the breastfeeding experience of their own wives! If their wives had had a difficult time or were unsuccessful then they legislated for difficulties with their patients and so put them off breastfeeding. A distinguished American paediatrician once lectured fellow paediatricians on infant feeding in New York. When by the end of his oration he still had not mentioned breast-feeding, one of the delegates asked why. The paediatrician answered that he never recommended breastfeeding because it was too difficult!

What help is there?
Pregnant women are often overwhelmed with help and advice from friends, relatives, neighbours and their medical advisers. The

doctor looking after the expectant mother may ask how she is going to feed her baby and may proffer some advice and even examine her breasts. When the baby is born, the midwife, obstetrician and paediatrician, together with friends, relatives and neighbours, will again offer advice about feeding the baby.

But although there may be masses of lay and professional 'help' and 'advice', because most people today have forgotten how to practise the art of successful breastfeeding, let alone how to teach it, such help may be of little or no value. It was exactly because of this confusion that self-help organisations came into being.

The National Childbirth Trust Breastfeeding Promotion Group has organised a network of mothers throughout Great Britain who have breastfed their children and have been trained as breastfeeding counsellors. They will help on the phone if you have problems and visit you at home if necessary.

La Leche League started when a small group of mothers realised that the only people who seemed to know what they were doing were other mothers who had breastfed their babies and had overcome problems on the way. La Leche League is now an international organisation whose slogan is 'Good mothering through breastfeeding'. Its groups hold meetings and discussions about breastfeeding and its group leaders give help on the phone or in person when necessary.

The Association of Breastfeeding Mothers is another, relatively new self-help organisation. If you have a problem with breastfeeding you need help there and then, before you give the baby that first bottle.

Your paediatrician may be helpful but he may not be as knowledgeable about how to breastfeed successfully as a trained mother whose main interest lies in helping other women to breastfeed.

Breastfeeding isn't always as easy as falling off a log, contrary to what many successful mothers will tell you. There's nothing more annoying than having to listen to people telling you how easy it is (and by implication what a failure you are if you are having trouble). We don't think breastfeeding is necessarily easy – it's often a lot harder than most women expect – especially in the early days.

If help is hard to come by, you can teach yourself how to cope successfully with problems and we'll show you how.

2 How breastfeeding works

This chapter and the next will give you an idea of how breastfeeding works and why breast milk is the best for your baby. The practical details of breastfeeding start in Chapter 6 but the next few chapters fill in the essential background knowledge you'll need to understand how to breastfeed and why things can go wrong. They'll bring you right up to date with all the major research carried out into breastfeeding over the last twenty years or so. It's an indictment of modern medicine that although a great deal of this key research has been published for years, many doctors and nurses are unaware of it.

Let's start by looking at the breasts themselves.

The breasts

A year or so before a girl's periods start, changes in the shape and size of her breasts, nipples and areolae begin and they carry on changing until her late teens. After this they remain the same (if her weight remains steady) until she becomes pregnant. Man is the only mammal in which the breasts enlarge before pregnancy. Breasts have also taken on a sexual role in courtship that isn't seen in other mammals and it's this that helps colour our attitudes to breast-feeding in the western world.

The breast is made up of fifteen to twenty segments, each containing glandular tissue leading to a main duct which opens at the nipple. This means that there are between fifteen and twenty ducts opening at the nipple. You can see these openings as little crevices and if you stop for a moment when you're feeding your baby, you'll see drops of milk coming from them. Sometimes you may see fine sprays of milk coming from several ducts at a time. Some ducts may merge within the nipple, so there may be fewer openings at the nipple than there are ducts.

In the pregnant or breastfeeding woman the glandular part of each segment of the breast is rather like a bunch of grapes on a stalk which is the milk duct. Each 'grape' is called an alveolus or milk gland and has a tiny duct leading to the 'stalk' or main duct. The milk gland is lined with milk-producing cells, each bordering on the little duct, so that milk produced by these cells goes from the small to the large ducts and thence to the nipples. Around each milk gland is a network of branching, star-like muscle cells (myo-epithelial cells) which can contract, so squeezing the milk gland and forcing milk from the cells into the ducts.

The main duct from each segment of the breast widens as it lies under the areola and is capable of further distension as it fills with milk. This means that just underneath the areola there are fifteen to twenty milk 'reservoirs'. The diameter of each of these when full can be between half and one centimetre, so it's easy to see that a lot of milk can be stored ready for the baby at the beginning of each feed. These reservoirs are capable of storing even more milk after several weeks of breastfeeding and some mothers notice that any leaking they may have had stops after six to eight weeks as their storage capacity increases.

The increase in size of the breasts during adolescence is caused by the laying down of fat and by the lengthening and branching of the milk ducts. At this stage there is very little true glandular tissue but the formation of buds which will later develop into the milk glands is now begun. All these changes are controlled by a woman's hormones.

During pregnancy many women notice tingling and fullness of their breasts as early as their first missed period. Indeed, breast sensations are often the first symptom of pregnancy. Little prominences around the areolae called Montgomery's tubercles become more noticeable at about six weeks. These tubercles have little glands in them that produce a substance that lubricates and protects the nipples during breastfeeding. Some women also produce milk from a tubercle and this is quite normal – anatomically they are like tiny breasts. By five months most women find they need a larger bra. In a first pregnancy, the nipples and areolae begin to darken now. If you lose your baby at any time after five months, you'll lactate just as if you had given birth at full term. All these changes are caused by hormones (some of which are present only in pregnancy) circulating in the blood. On average, each breast weighs one and a half pounds more at the end of pregnancy, mainly because of the development of glandular tissue and the proliferation of the milk ducts.

The size of your breasts before pregnancy will have no bearing on your ability to breastfeed because some small breasts actually contain more milk-producing glands than do larger ones. It's the *increase* in the size of your breasts during pregnancy that is a good indicator of your ability to feed easily. As a general rule, if you need a bra one or two sizes larger by the end of pregnancy, you should have little trouble getting off to a good start. It has been found that the younger a woman is when she has her first pregnancy, the greater is the increase in the size of her breasts. This may explain why it is that, with women having their first babies, younger ones tend to produce more milk than older ones at first. Women with very small breasts may be at a slight disadvantage early on because their breasts can become overfilled more quickly than larger breasts and so either leak or have to be offered to the baby more frequently. As their storage capacity increases over the first few weeks this becomes less of a problem.

While we're on the subject of breast size, it's interesting to note that mothers often comment on the size of their babies' breasts. Newborn babies often have enlarged breasts. This is because of maternal hormones travelling across the placenta before birth. Sometimes milk even comes out of a baby's breasts. This is often called witches' milk and is seen in both boys and girls. The treatment is to ignore it – it will eventually disappear.

Not only do a woman's nipples become larger during pregnancy but they also become more protractile (able to be lengthened), and so easier for the baby to take hold of with his mouth. There are a few women whose nipples don't change like this and their babies may have problems in 'latching on' at first. Details of how to overcome this problem can be found on pages 74–5.

Milk production
Production of milk by the milk glands is under the influence of the hormones prolactin, growth hormone, the corticosteroids, thyroxine and insulin. Each milk gland is surrounded by a fine network of blood vessels and it is through this blood supply that the hormones reach the milk-producing cells. Blood also provides the

materials from which milk is actually made by the cells.

Prolactin is the main milk-producing hormone and appears from the eighth week of pregnancy onwards, reaching its peak with the birth of the baby. It is prevented from producing milk in any volume during pregnancy by the high levels of oestrogen made by the placenta. After the baby is born and with the loss of the placenta, the oestrogen 'brakes' are removed and prolactin starts milk production in earnest. This usually occurs between the second and fourth days but the milk can come in earlier in women feeding their babies frequently and in an unrestricted way from birth and in those having their second or subsequent babies. Usually the milk comes in slowly but it may come in a deluge. This is quite normal, so don't let it worry you. The way to cope with it is to encourage your baby to feed as often as you need to keep you comfortable.

Prolactin, the hormone that 'turns on the taps', is produced by the pituitary gland in the brain. The most important factor in the continued release of prolactin is nipple stimulation which sends nervous impulses to the pituitary. The holding and squeezing of the nipple and areola by the baby's mouth are a more important factor in nipple stimulation than his sucking. Nipple stimulation increases the mother's prolactin which in turn increases her milk supply, so the more the baby is at the breast, the more milk is produced. Prolactin levels fluctuate throughout the day and are highest at night, even in non-lactating women.

As milk is produced by the milk glands, it is secreted into the milk ducts. We've already seen that the parts of the ducts under the areolae are capable of storing milk. This milk, known as foremilk, is low in fat content and hence in calories. Every woman produces milk after childbirth and so will have foremilk available for her baby whenever he wants to feed. However, the bulk of the milk (the hindmilk) is stored in the milk glands at any one time and is supplied only if the *let-down reflex* operates.

Getting milk into a baby in large enough amounts is a skill that needs to be learnt but like most skills it's acquired all the more quickly if you know the mechanisms involved. There are two vital mechanisms: one is the let-down reflex we've just mentioned and the other is the law of demand and supply. Let's look at each in turn.

The let-down reflex

After a feed, the milk-producing cells in the milk glands gradually enlarge, becoming round and full as they produce more milk. The fullness and slight lumpiness you may feel some time after a feed is caused by these swollen milk glands with their laden cells and ducts.

The milk in the cells can be forced into the ducts very quickly by the contraction of the muscle cells surrounding each milk gland and when this happens the milk is said to have been let down. This is the only way in which the baby can immediately get this milk: without the let-down, the milk stays in the milk glands and the baby drinks only the foremilk.

Milk released by the let-down is known as hindmilk. Hindmilk is rich in calories and fat and without it a baby will not get enough milk to thrive. Foremilk contains 10 calories/ounce and hindmilk 30 calories/ounce.

With the let-down, milk is pushed into the ducts so quickly that it may spray or drip from the nipples. This occurs in a series of spurts with a gap between each. There may be several let-downs during each feed.

The reason that many women fail to breastfeed successfully is that their let-down reflex is faulty. This reflex is a delicately balanced mechanism, especially in the early weeks after childbirth when external factors can prevent its satisfactory development and action. When you hear people talking about the 'establishment' of breastfeeding, they are really talking about the establishment of a satisfactory, reliable, well-conditioned let-down reflex.

The main factor involved is the stimulation of the skin of the nipple and the tissues under the areola which normally occurs when the baby is suckled at the breast. This is the same stimulus that causes prolactin release. Nervous impulses travel from the nipple to the pituitary gland and cause the release of another hormone – oxytocin – into the blood. Oxytocin is taken in the blood to the breast and makes the muscle cells around the milk glands squeeze milk into the ducts. This cycle – of suckling; nervous messages to the pituitary; oxytocin release; contraction of muscle cells with the subsequent release of milk into the ducts – is what is known as the let-down reflex.

The time taken for the let-down reflex to work varies from woman to woman and in any one woman it can vary from day to day according to her surroundings, emotional state and other factors. When a baby is put to the breast the let-down takes a minimum of thirty to fifty seconds to work but it often takes longer than this and it can take two to three minutes of nipple stimulation for the maximum milk flow to be produced.

This means that a hungry baby may have finished all the available foremilk before any hindmilk has been let down and this delay can make him frustrated. Such frustration can worry the inexperienced mother to such an extent that she doesn't let down her milk at all. The let-down can be such a delicate mechanism that emotions such as fear, worry and embarrassment can prevent its action.

Nipple stimulation is not the only way in which the milk can be let down – the reflex is easily conditioned by other stimuli. The sight, sound or thought of your baby (or even someone else's baby) can suddenly let down your milk, particularly if you haven't fed for some time. Some women find that as they prepare to feed their babies, their let-down works before suckling is begun at all, simply because the reflex has been conditioned by their routine. This is a good thing because the baby then doesn't have to wait for the milk to flow.

Besides causing the let-down, oxytocin has other effects. The uterus is sensitive to oxytocin and may contract when there is an increased level in the blood. The uterine contractions are rhythmical and are the cause of the 'afterpains' some mothers feel while feeding in the first few days. Also, while the milk is being let down, the breasts may tingle and feel tense. The let-down is usually a pleasant feeling for the mother and has been described as 'something between a sneeze and an orgasm'.

At the same time as the milk is let down, the skin of the breasts feels warmer to the touch than usual. In the early days of feeding it's easy to know when your let-down reflex is working because of the sensations in the breasts, leaking (dripping or spraying) of milk from the breasts, the warmth of the breast skin and the contractions of the womb. Some mothers have none of these sensations yet have a very good let-down reflex – and any given woman may experience different let-down sensations from baby to baby. Other women report that the feelings they experience as their milk is let down change or even disappear completely throughout the months of breastfeeding. One mother described a sensation of cold water trickling down behind her breastbone when her milk was let down in the first few weeks of breastfeeding. This was later replaced by a tingling feeling throughout her breasts and, later still, by an itching sensation beneath her areolae. Many women say that the removal of the milk by the sucking of the baby gives a very welcome feeling of relief as the tension in the full breast is lessened.

Leaking

Warmth from a hot bath or from your baby's mouth can cause initial leaking of milk without a true let-down. This is because there are contractile muscle fibres in the nipple and areola which are normally held contracted, so keeping the ducts closed. Warmth lengthens these fibres and releases their tight hold on the ducts, allowing milk to escape. If the breasts are full of milk, simply leaning forward or to one side can cause leaking.

So far we've only considered the milk-producing effects of the mother's hormones but they also have other effects. The hormones produced during lactation seem to give the breastfeeding mother a special feeling of happiness and an ability to relax. Animal research has shown that lactating rats are actually buffered against stressful situations by their hormones and it's quite possible that this may also be true in humans. Some people go so far as to call prolactin the 'mothering hormone' or the 'happiness hormone'.

How the baby gets the milk

So much for the production and let-down of milk but how does it actually get to the baby? There are many old wives' tales about suckling but the most common is that the baby gets the milk by sucking. Actually, the baby gets the milk from the breast by a combination of *three* methods: sucking, milking and just allowing let-down milk (or leaking milk from a full breast) to drip or spray into his mouth. The sucking reflex (see also page 175) is instinctive and is strongest 20–30 minutes after birth, which is why a baby should be put to the breast in the first half hour after birth. Thereafter it becomes temporarily much weaker if the baby hasn't been put to the breast. After forty hours it gets stronger again. While at the breast, the baby exerts suction to keep the nipple and areola in his mouth and in so doing will suck in some milk. He gets the foremilk from the reservoirs under the areola by a 'milking' action of his jaws. The further he can draw the nipple and areola into his mouth, the better he'll be able to empty the reservoirs. This is why the protractility of the nipples is so important. This milking action stimulates the let-down reflex which ejects milk from the nipple in fine jets so that all he has to do is swallow. You'll notice that your baby will take several gulps of milk in a row and then rest for a while, keeping the breast in his mouth, before taking more gulps. This is because the milk lets down in spurts with a gap between each spurt. If oxytocin levels in the blood are continuously monitored during a feed they can be seen to rise and fall in waves corresponding with the ejection of the milk.

The swallowing reflex is essential for the baby to get the milk from his mouth to his stomach. All three of the reflexes seen in breastfeeding babies – the rooting reflex (see page 82), the sucking reflex and the swallowing reflex – may be temporarily absent in pre-term babies or impaired in babies who are brain damaged, jaundiced or who have an infection. Mechanical problems such as a cleft palate may also interfere with them.

Demand and supply

All the time a baby is feeding, the nipple and surrounding area are stimulated, so causing the pituitary gland to release prolactin and oxytocin. Since prolactin controls milk production it's easy to see that the more suckling there is, the more prolactin will be produced, which in turn produces more milk. Also, the more episodes of suckling there are, the more reliable the let-down reflex becomes. This is the basis of the second mechanism of successful breast-feeding – that of demand and supply. If those caring for new mothers understood this principle, there would be far fewer breast-feeding failures.

'Supply and demand' would not be a good term because the demand produces the supply and not the other way round. The more feeds your baby 'asks for' and gets in a day, the greater the supply of milk there will be. This has been proven in many surveys. For instance, in one survey in Sheffield as long ago as 1952, demand-fed babies gained weight faster than those fed according to a schedule, showing that their mothers were producing more milk by feeding more often.

There are no limits to the number of feeds you can give your baby. Every time he asks, he should be fed. This doesn't mean to say, though, that you can feed your baby only when he asks for a feed. If you want to feed him because your breasts are full, because you want the pleasure of cuddling him at your breast, or because it is a convenient time for you, do.

Successful or natural breastfeeding puts no rules or limits on suckling time (see page 86).

Babies allowed to feed as often as they want take very variable numbers of feeds during the twenty-four hours. In the early days some babies may want feeding every hour or so and the greatest number of feeds often occurs on the fifth day after birth. In the Sheffield survey we've just mentioned, 29 per cent of babies fed on demand wanted eight feeds on the fifth day and 10 per cent wanted more than nine.

In a textbook for doctors published in 1906, when successful breastfeeding was the norm, the following schedule of feeds was recommended:

First day	4 feeds
Second day	6 feeds
Rest of the first month	10 feeds
Second and third months	8 feeds
Fourth and fifth months	7 feeds
Sixth to eleventh months	6 feeds

This is a far cry from the schedules so often recommended for breastfed babies in hospitals today (every four hours for a large baby and every three hours for a small one). This sort of schedule produces notoriously poor results whereas the 1906 type was much more successful. *However, completely unrestricted, natural breastfeeding involving very frequent feeds in the early days is best of all, and any schedule should be discarded by the mother who wants to breastfeed successfully.*

A survey in Africa throws interesting light on this subject. Researchers watched mothers sleeping with their babies over many nights to see how often the babies fed while their mothers slept. No baby went longer than twenty minutes without feeding! Contrast these lucky babies with western babies who are usually rationed to one feed a night until their mother's milk dries up completely.

One sure way of reducing the number of feeds your baby asks for (and thus reducing the amount of stimulation your breasts get and hence your chances of breastfeeding successfully) is to keep your baby apart from you. In countries where babies are carried by their mothers by day and lie next to them at night, and where few clothes are worn by mother or baby, the babies spend very much more time at their mother's breasts than do Western babies. It's not surprising that those babies who are allowed virtually unrestricted access to their mother's breasts are almost always breastfed fully and successfully for many months. The supply of milk doesn't dry up quickly but continues for an average of three years until the baby no longer wants to be at the breast.

Never compare your baby with that of your neighbour. Each baby is unique and should be allowed to be so. Some settle into a routine of six feeds a day within a few weeks but this is certainly *not* a goal to be aimed for, it's just one of many patterns that your baby may adopt in time. A word of warning here – one leading authority in the UK has said that in her experience if a baby has five or fewer feeds in a day, the likelihood is that the mother's milk will have dried up in a month through lack of stimulation of the breasts. *However many feeds your baby wants, let him have them.*

The length of a feed is also a matter for the individual baby to decide and shouldn't be laid down by doctors, midwives or even mothers. The average feeding time at one breast is about ten minutes but there are some babies who get all they need in five minutes and yet others who need twenty minutes or much more at each breast before they are satisfied. Feeding times vary for several reasons. First, the let-down may be slow to work so the baby doesn't start getting hindmilk for two or three minutes. Second, some babies are much greedier than others, suck more strongly and so get all they need in a shorter time. Third, some babies – especially in the early days – may not be very alert and so will need to take their time over a feed. All these situations are discussed in more detail later.

Though we have been conditioned into talking about the periods of time a baby spends at the breast as 'feeds', it would be far more helpful if we could forget this concept because it inevitably makes us think of a baby's 'feed' purely as a mealtime – a time to get the milk down in as businesslike a way as possible. Many babies, however – especially in the early days – like to drink their milk in a very leisurely, long-drawn-out way, snoozing between bouts of sucking. While snoozing, they may let go of the breast only to wake again in a short while, or they may hold the nipple in their mouth and give an occasional gentle, 'fluttering' sort of suck for minutes at a time. It's not uncommon for a young baby sometimes to spend hours at the breast in this fashion if he is allowed to. Such behaviour, which is perfectly normal, makes the counting of feeds quite meaningless. It's not difficult to understand that the baby allowed to behave like this is stimulating the breast much more than the baby allowed only a certain number of 'proper' feeds of a certain length.

It's important not to curtail the length of feeds in the first few days particularly, because it's all too easy to take the baby from the breast before the let-down has worked at all. Many hospitals insist on very short suckling times in the first few days to prevent sore nipples but as we'll see later this is a fallacious argument. Short suckling times often prevent or delay the establishment of successful lactation and are of absolutely no benefit to mother or baby.

Finally, a question often asked by mothers who don't want to breastfeed is how they can dry up their milk. Today we know that there is no need for any drugs to do this. If a mother simply doesn't breastfeed, her milk will eventually dry up by itself. Oestrogens, once used to dry up milk, can have side-effects such as venous thrombosis, and stopping the drug often causes a rebound of milk production. The use of new drugs such as bromocriptine to dry up milk is not only unnecessary but also expensive.

One other advantage of not using drugs to dry up milk artificially is that if a mother changes her mind and decides to breastfeed, it is much easier for her to work up her milk supply than if it had been artificially suppressed.

So much for the breasts themselves – now let's look at the milk they produce.

3 Breast milk – the perfect food

Until very recently it was thought that the advantages of breast milk were few. To most medical and nursing students these advantages were usually summed up as follows:

1 it's at the right temperature;
2 it contains exactly what the baby needs;
3 it's bacteria-free;
4 it comes in such cute containers; and
5 the cat can't get at it!

For years this was the sort of level at which doctors and nurses were taught to consider breast milk. Small wonder then that, when the baby milk manufacturers came up with their modified, 'improved' milks, both mothers and the medical profession thought they were getting something every bit as good as breast milk – and perhaps even better.

Other mammals' milk

The outstanding characteristic of mammals is that they suckle or feed their young with their milk at least until their young can get their own food. As mammals are so different from one another, it's not surprising that the milk they produce differs too. If an elephant, a rat, a sheep, a whale and a human ate similar diets, it might be reasonable to expect that the milk they produced for their young would be similar. But of course they don't and their milks are correspondingly different. Over scores of thousands of years each mammal has developed a milk to suit its own young. This milk takes into account the animal's rate of growth, type of digestive tract, body composition and many other factors.

The basic similarity that runs through all milks, though, is that they are made up of the same groups of substances: water, proteins, fats, carbohydrates, minerals, vitamins, anti-infective substances, hormones, live cells, enzymes and other factors. The differences occur because these substances are present in different amounts and in varying proportions. In addition to this, these eleven things are not single entities (apart from water) but are often made up of whole families of substances, each one different from the next. For example, there are many different sorts of fats, some of which differ from woman to woman, let alone between woman and cow!

When we look at whale milk we find it has a very high fat content, which in turn gives it a very high calorie content. (It is in fact richer than double cream.) This is essential because the infant whale has to form a layer of thick blubber very quickly so as to protect it from the cold water. The protein content of rabbits' milk is very high compared with human milk. It contains 14 per cent protein compared with the 1.2 per cent in human milk. This is necessary because the growth rate of the young rabbit is so fast. (A rabbit doubles its birth weight in six days, whereas a human baby takes about 140 days.) High milk protein levels are a must for every newborn mammal that grows quickly, because protein provides the basic building blocks for the growth of body tissues. Compared with most other mammalian young, human babies grow very slowly and breast milk has a correspondingly lower level of protein.

Over the years there have been reports of mammals taking the young of other species into their care and feeding them but this is very unusual. The first time one group of mammals used another's milk to any great extent was when humans started to give their babies cows' milk this century. Of course, over the centuries the occasional baby has been reared on the milk of another animal (Romulus and Remus were supposedly reared by a wolf) but the widespread use of cows' milk is a new phenomenon. Before this century if a mother didn't want to feed her baby, another woman had to take over if the baby was to have a good chance of surviving, and in some countries even today a baby will die if the mother doesn't feed it herself.

Why did we choose cows' milk as our breast milk substitute? It's a particularly good question because cows' milk is by no means the nearest in composition to human milk – donkey milk is much closer! People in other countries have used the milk from goats, donkeys, buffalo, sheep, llamas, reindeer, mares and camels for their babies over the years but the great move towards artificial feeding came from the West where herds of cows were already being reared for meat and dairy produce, so it seemed convenient and economically sensible to use cows' milk. Cows are also docile, easily herded animals that produce large volumes of milk from a given volume of grass. Add to this the fact that their four teats make for easy milking and it soon becomes clear why we have tended to use cows as a source of milk.

The most obvious differences between cows' milk and breast milk are that cows' milk contains more protein and less sugar. This led doctors and food scientists to 'modify' it earlier this century so that it came to resemble breast milk more closely. They did this by diluting it and adding sugar. This basic modification was used for years and mothers either adapted liquid cows' milk by diluting it with water, adding sugar and boiling it, or they bought dried, evaporated or condensed milk and made up their own formula by adding water and sugar in the recommended amounts. Over the years we have come to realise that these basic modifications are not enough because of the many differences between the two milks. We now know that these differences can lead to medical problems in babies drinking cows' milk preparations and we'll consider some of these later.

What milk contains
Water
The liquid part of milk is water and all the other constituents are either dissolved or suspended in it, making it appear white, creamy or yellow, depending on the proportions of the various substances present.

Water is vital for the existence of every cell in the body and a lack of it causes dehydration, cell damage and, eventually, death. Certain body cells are more susceptible than others to dehydration and brain cells are especially at risk. A dehydrated baby runs the risk of brain damage.

Breast milk is the perfect food for human babies because the proportions of water and the other constituents are just right. Many mothers worry that their milk might be too 'watery'. This is very unlikely and anyway there's nothing you can tell about the nutritional value of breast milk simply by looking at it. Yellowish breast milk is in no way superior to thin, bluish-white milk nor is it comparable to rich, creamy cows' milk.

A thirsty baby given enough breast milk gets the right amount of water to satisfy his thirst. A breastfed baby need never be given water, provided he gets enough breast milk. In very hot weather the breastfeeding *mother* should drink more water, not the baby. On the other hand a baby drinking cows' milk is in danger of taking too high a proportion of the substances dissolved in the water because the concentrations of some of them are relatively high (even in modified cows' milk). This is especially likely to happen if he is already dehydrated from diarrhoea, vomiting, or sweating from a fever, unless he is given additional water.

In addition to these unavoidable hazards mothers sometimes make up milk feeds too strong. Recent modifications of cows' milk preparations have helped to some extent but the proportions of water and other substances are still by no means the same as those of breast milk and there's still some danger in over-strong feeds, especially in the early weeks of life.

The stools of bottle-fed babies contain less water than those of breastfed babies and this is one reason why they get constipated more often.

Protein

About 1.2 per cent of breast milk is protein. This protein is made up of curd protein (casein) and the whey proteins (lactalbumin and lactoglobulin). Cows' milk has 3.3 per cent protein (a calf doubles its birth weight in fifty days) and this extra is composed of six times as much casein as there is in human milk.

When milk enters a baby's stomach, it's turned into curds and whey. The curds are made of casein, so it's not surprising that the curds of cows' milk are much bulkier than those of breast milk. They are so tough and bulky that many babies get indigestion if they are given unmodified cows' milk to drink.

This is the main reason behind the basic 'modification' of cows' milk – dilution with water. Adding water dilutes the tough, indigestible casein. Boiling, homogenisation and the addition of various chemicals have also been used to alter the casein so as to make it less tough and indigestible.

Breast milk protein forms finely separated curds in the stomach which then pass quickly and easily through into the small intestine where they are easily broken down. This means that the stomach of a breastfed baby empties more quickly than that of a bottle-fed baby and this is why he gets hungry more quickly and needs more frequent feeds. Cows' milk curds stay in the stomach for about four hours but breast milk leaves the stomach in about one and a half hours. *So four-hourly feeding for a bottle-fed baby is reasonable, but a breastfed baby will need feeding more often.*

A baby uses only about half the protein available in cows' milk, whilst a breastfed baby uses all the protein in breast milk, with virtually no wastage. The protein a bottle-fed baby doesn't use is partly passed out in the stools (which makes a bottle-fed baby's stools bulkier than a breastfed baby's) and partly broken down before being excreted by the kidneys in the urine. Because there is so little wastage from breast milk, a baby has to drink less of it. This is why breastfed babies normally drink a much smaller volume than do bottle-fed ones. Test weighing a breastfed baby can easily be misleading if this is forgotten – *the amount a breastfed baby drinks should never be compared with the amount drunk by a bottle-fed one.*

The lactoglobulin fraction of milk protein contains highly specialised proteins – the immunoglobulins (IgA, IgD, IgE, IgG and IgM). These carry antibodies against disease and recent research into these substances has revolutionised our thinking on breast milk. For years it was thought that a baby obtained antibodies from its mother only before birth across the placenta and that none were given via breast milk. That this was not the only method of antibody transfer in other mammals had been known for a long time. We now know that babies continue to receive these essential antibodies from their mothers' milk – assuming of course that they're breastfed. Colostrum, the first milk produced in pregnancy and in the first few days after birth, contains large amounts of lactoglobulin, which is one reason why we can now say with complete assurance that colostrum is vitally important for the health of a baby. Mature breast milk also contains antibodies but in smaller amounts than those in colostrum.

These milk antibodies are similar to those which the mother has in her blood and protect the baby to some extent against bacterial and viral illnesses from which the mother has suffered or has been immunised against. They can act locally in the baby's gut and can also be absorbed into his bloodstream through the gut lining. Among the illnesses that a baby can be protected from in this way (though to a varying and unpredictable extent) are tetanus, whooping cough, pneumonia, diphtheria, *E. coli* gastroenteritis, typhoid, dysentery, flu and various other viral illnesses including polio. Later a baby will manufacture his own antibodies in response to infection or immunisation but during the first few months he can't and so has to get antibodies from his mother. This period of absent and then gradually increasing antibody formation by the baby has been called the 'immunity gap' and it's a gap that can be filled only by breast milk.

Because a mother has had an infection, that *doesn't* mean that her breastfed baby will definitely be protected against it, though there may be complete or partial protection.

Immunoglobulin A (IgA) in the mother's colostrum and milk coats the lining of the baby's gut in the first few days after birth and prevents many infective organisms and other large protein molecules from entering the baby's bloodstream. When the baby begins to make his own IgA, his mother's becomes unnecessary but in the meantime this IgA coating prevents the development not only of some generalised infections but also of allergy to various foodstuffs in many babies. We'll talk about this more in Chapter 4.

Cows' milk contains antibodies too but of course these are antibodies against cows' diseases, not human ones. In any case lactoglobulin (together with lactoferrin, another anti-infective agent) is altered to such an extent by the heating involved in the treatment of fresh cows' milk that it loses its antibody activity. So the cows' milk preparations available to human babies don't contain active antibodies and even if they did these wouldn't be of any use! The ultimate irony is that calves reared on heat-treated milk or on dried milk powder get more enteritis than those drinking fresh untreated milk. This enteritis is effectively treated by giving them fresh cows' milk. The reason that even calves fare badly on treated cows' milk is that this treatment destroys the milk's antibody activity.

An interesting parallel to this was seen in a nursery in Belgrade where an epidemic of *E. coli* gastroenteritis could not be stopped even when the previously bottle-fed babies were all fed with donated breast milk (boiled before use). Not until the breast milk was given fresh from the donors, with no boiling, was the epidemic controlled.

Besides protein in milk there are free amino acids and the proportions of these differ in human and cows' milk. Breast milk, for instance, contains more cystine compared with cows' milk which contains more of another amino acid known as methionine. This is especially important for premature babies because they are incapable of using methionine until they become more mature.

Nucleotides are building blocks necessary for protein manufacture (like the amino acids) and they are present in human milk in larger amounts than in cows' milk. More important perhaps is the fact that the main one found in cows' milk, orotic acid, is not found at all in human milk. More research needs to be done before we know how important this is. But it raises a crucial question. Might there actually be substances in cows' milk that, although present only in tiny amounts, could be positively harmful to human babies?

Fat

In a well-nourished woman the fat in her milk reflects the composition of the fat in her diet. If a mother has an inadequate calorie intake the pattern of fatty acids in her milk is similar to that of the fat stores under her skin. Milk fat is present in both saturated and unsaturated forms. Breast milk contains a higher percentage of unsaturated fat than does cows' milk. This recently led some baby milk manufacturers to replace some of the fat in cows' milk with unsaturated vegetable oils in an attempt to make the milk more like breast milk. Their early efforts led to some dire consequences as linoleic acid (one of these unsaturated vegetable oils) was added in far greater quantities than are naturally present in human milk. Some babies suffered from a severe kind of anaemia as a result.

Whilst cows' milk contains less linoleic acid than breast milk, most baby milks contain enough to prevent the symptoms of deficiency (poor growth and thick scaly skin) even without the substitution of vegetable oils.

As yet we don't know whether the unsaturated fat content of breast milk is in any way protective against heart disease. This is still a matter for speculation. We do know though that another essential body fat – cholesterol – is present in larger amounts in breast milk than in cows' milk. After all the scares surrounding cholesterol and heart attacks and the possible link between the two you might well ask whether a cholesterol-rich milk is best for babies.

Ironically, it looks as though the higher cholesterol levels somehow accustom breastfed babies to handling cholesterol. This is thought to stand them in good stead for the future and might even prevent or reduce the likelihood of later heart disease (see Chapter 4).

Fats are split into simpler fatty substances in the gut by naturally occurring enzymes called lipases. The digestion of cows' milk fat (butterfat) by lipase leads to the release of a fatty acid, palmitic acid, which combines with calcium in the gut and is passed out in the stools, so robbing the body of calcium. In human milk, palmitic acid is built into the fat particles in such a way that when fat is digested by lipase, the acid is not released as a free fatty acid but is absorbed into the bloodstream together with part of the broken-down fat particle. In this way calcium is not lost. This is important because when babies are growing fast (and a baby grows at its fastest on the very first day of its life) they need a plentiful supply of calcium to build strong bones and teeth.

Human milk contains some lipase of its own, unlike cows' milk which relies solely on lipase in the baby's intestine for its digestion. The fat in breast milk starts being digested by the milk lipase even before it reaches the gut. This means that some of the valuable fatty acids are available for use sooner than would be the case with cows' milk. Fat provides more than 50 per cent of the energy provided by mature breast milk.

Fat is necessary for the body's development in many ways but it is especially important for the development of the outer coating of the nerves. It seems likely that the specific pattern of fatty acids in human milk has developed in such a way as to supply the rapidly growing brain and nerves with exactly the right building materials at the right time – early infancy – when these tissues grow faster than at any other time.

Less important but of more practical significance to the mother is the fact that if a breastfed baby regurgitates any milk, the smell is not particularly unpleasant, whereas a bottle-fed baby's vomit has a characteristically foul, sour smell which quickly permeates the clothing of both mother and child. The difference is due to the presence of fatty acid – butyric acid – in cows' milk, which smells unpleasant when partially digested.

Carbohydrates

Both breast milk and cows' milk contain lactose (milk sugar) but breast milk has more of it. Lactose is split into two parts in the gut – galactose and glucose. Galactose is an essential ingredient of the myelin coatings of nerve fibres and can also be synthesised in the liver from glucose. The old practice of diluting cows' milk and adding ordinary sugar (sucrose) meant that dietary galactose was in short supply to the bottle-fed baby. Some of the more recent modifications of cows' milk have included adding lactose instead of sucrose.

Breast milk also contains glucose and some other sugars which are completely absent or present in much lower quantities in cows' milk.

It's interesting that certain sugars (the oligosaccharides) vary according to the mother's blood group.

The bifidus factor is another carbohydrate present in breast milk but virtually absent from cows' milk. This is a very valuable protective factor against infection in the gut, as we'll see later in the chapter.

Minerals

Whole cows' milk (unmodified) contains almost four times as many minerals as breast milk, which is one reason why a baby's kidneys might be overworked if he were fed on whole cows' milk.

Modified cows' milk has much lower levels of minerals but even so there is no milk available which has the low mineral level of breast milk. It is possible to lower the levels of the minerals in cows' milk further by a process called demineralisation but there is a big snag to this. We don't know how many useful though unknown minerals are completely removed whilst reducing the levels of the ones we know exist. We just don't know the exact contents of cows' or breast milk.

As minerals are so important to the health of a baby, we'll discuss some of them in more detail.

Sodium The level in breast milk is ideal for human babies. The level in modified cows' milk is lower than in fresh cows' milk but is still higher than in breast milk. Sodium is closely linked with water in the body and an imbalance of either can be serious and even fatal. This is why so much care must be taken of babies who are bottle-fed if they develop any illness such as diarrhoea, vomiting or a fever (which all reduce their water level) and why so much care must be taken not to prepare feeds which are too strong (so increasing their salt level).

Calcium, phosphorus and magnesium Higher levels of all these are present in cows' milk, though modification reduces them to some extent. Several problems are known to have arisen from this in the past, including a type of muscular spasm known as neonatal tetany, convulsions, and poor development of the enamel of the teeth, followed by severe dental decay.

Iron This is one mineral present in larger amounts (twice as much) in breast milk as in unmodified cows' milk, though the levels in modified cows' milk are higher than in breast milk. Recent research indicates that the iron in breast milk is better absorbed into the bloodstream than that in cows' milk formulae. Certain substances such as vitamins C and E and copper help iron to be absorbed more efficiently and these are present in higher amounts in breast milk. We know that the addition of iron to milk can reduce the anti-infective properties of lactoferrin, so the low levels of iron in breast milk should not be seen as inferior to the higher levels in modified cows' milk. The totally breastfed baby almost never becomes anaemic.

Fluoride See page 46.

Trace elements
These include copper, zinc, manganese, chromium, cobalt, molybdenum, selenium and iodine. There are fifteen trace elements known to be essential for a baby and most are part of enzymes.

Vitamins
Breast milk contains more vitamins A, C and E than cows' milk but less vitamin K. In mothers well nourished during pregnancy and having a well-balanced diet while breastfeeding, there is no evidence that their fully breastfed babies normally need any vitamin supplements in the first six months of life. Some doctors still recommend that breastfed babies should have vitamin D supplements but this stems from the earlier and incorrect assumption that

breast milk contained less of the vitamin than did cows' milk. Recent research has shown that there is water soluble vitamin D in breast milk besides the fat-soluble fraction that we already knew about, and that there is more of this in human milk than in cows' milk. Sunshine is a far better source of vitamin D than any food. Vitamin D produced in the skin after exposure to sunlight can be stored and used during the winter months. It makes sense for the woman who is pregnant or breastfeeding to get as much sun as she can and for babies to be allowed to sunbathe when possible, taking care to avoid overexposure.

Although sunshine is the most important source of vitamin D, it's sensible to ensure that your diet during pregnancy and breast-feeding includes plenty of vitamin D-containing foods (such as margarine, fatty fish, eggs and butter). For mothers who have little exposure to sunlight or whose diets are deficient in this vitamin, vitamin D supplements are recommended.

The baby of a mother who is healthy and eating well will not need extra vitamin C. Research shows that a mother's vitamin C is concentrated in her breast milk so as to ensure that the baby gets enough. Even women who have scurvy do not produce babies deficient in vitamin C. If the mother's diet is deficient in this vitamin, *she* will need supplements of vitamin C.

Vitamin C passes readily from a mother's serum into her milk. If a food or drink containing vitamin C is taken, the level in the milk rises within half an hour.

Now to vitamin K. Although breast milk contains less of this vitamin than does cows' milk, there is no reason to suppose that breastfed babies should normally suffer from a lack of it. To prevent a possible shortage of vitamin K in the newborn (which causes bleeding) some babies in the UK are given an injection of vitamin K after birth, whether or not the mother is going to breastfeed.

In general, the principle should be to give any additional foods and vitamins necessary for the baby's well-being to the *mother* and not to the baby direct. If a mother's nutrition is good then she'll pass on all the right nutrients in her breast milk in the perfect proportions for her baby.

Anti-infective factors

We've already talked about the antibodies in breast milk but there are other substances which also help fight infection in the baby and many of these are more plentiful and more active in breast milk than in cows' milk.

The very proportion of the food substances in breast milk compared with those in cows' milk prevents the growth of certain organisms such as *E. coli* and dysentery and typhoid bacteria in the baby's gut. The high lactose, low phosphorus and low protein levels in particular do this.

The breastfed baby's gut, like that of the bottle-fed baby, contains thousands of tiny organisms. These are of an entirely different kind in the bottle-fed baby, though, and account for the foul smell of a bottle-fed baby's stools compared with the sweet smell of the stools of a breastfed baby. The organisms in the breastfed baby are members of the *Lactobacillus bifidus* family and are encouraged to grow by a special nitrogen-containing sugar – *the bifidus factor* – which is not present in useful amounts in cows' milk. The lactobacilli produce acetic and lactic acids which together prevent the growth of many disease-producing organisms such as *E. coli* (a common cause of gastroenteritis in the bottle-fed baby), the dysentery bacillus and the yeasts which cause thrush. There is also a possibility that the bifidus factor itself interferes with the flu virus.

An important anti-infective factor in breast milk present in much greater amounts (ten or twenty times more) than in cows' milk is the protein *lactoferrin*. Together with one of the immunoglobulins (IgA), lactoferrin inhibits the growth of many organisms, including *E. coli*, yeasts and staphylococci, by robbing them of the iron they need for growth. An important discovery is that extra iron prevents this action because the organisms then have enough to use to grow and divide. So giving a breastfed baby iron supplements may encourage infections of the gut. To any mother whose baby has had gastroenteritis this is far from an academic argument! Lactoferrin, like antibodies, loses its activity when milk is boiled, so the small amount that is present in cows' milk is useless in baby milk preparations.

Three more factors interact with each other to kill bacteria: *lysozyme*, present in breast milk in amounts 300 times greater than in cows' milk; *immunoglobulin A*; and a substance called *complement*. Lysozyme is present in other body secretions such as tears, where it helps prevent infections of the eyes and eyelids. The level of lysozyme falls in the first few months of a baby's life, then it starts rising, until at six months there is more than there was in colostrum. At a year there is even more.

Breast milk also contains an *anti-staphylococcal factor*; *hydrogen peroxide* and *vitamin C* which together kill bacteria such as *E. coli*; an enzyme *lactoperoxidase* which inhibits the growth of bacteria; and many *live cells*.

These live cells are white cells similar to some of those in the bloodstream. This means that breast milk is a living fluid, unlike cows' milk preparations (by the time they reach the baby, when all the cells have been killed by processing). The lymphoid cells in breast milk make IgA as well as an anti-viral substance called *interferon*. These cells can also be absorbed from the gut into the bloodstream of the baby where they continue their work of making immunoglobulins. Other cells in breast milk are called macrophages. These are large cells which can actively engulf particles such as bacteria and also produce lactoferrin, lysozyme and complement. Neutrophils and epithelial cells are also present.

Other substances which are not antibodies and yet act against certain viruses such as the polio, mumps and encephalitis viruses have been found in breast milk.

An interesting new field of research lies with certain viral infections of the mother such as cytomegalovirus or rubella infection. It is thought that such viruses in breast milk may give the baby an infection which – because of the antibodies – is very mild. The baby is virtually being immunised by the breast milk against his mother's infection.

Hormones

Many hormones have been found in breast milk, including prostaglandins, insulin, gonadotropin-releasing hormone, thyroid-releasing hormone, thyroid-stimulating hormone, prolactin, gonadotropins, ovarian steroids, corticosteroids, erythropoietin, parathyroid hormone and thyroid hormones (T_3 and T_4). At one time the maternal thyroid hormones in breast milk were thought to protect hypothyroid babies, but are no longer considered sufficient. Hypothyroidism should be detected and treated as soon as possible however the baby is being fed.

Some of these hormones, for instance the prostaglandins, are not found at all in cows' milk formula. Their importance to the baby is as yet largely unknown, though research is in progress. Among other important functions, prostaglandins may help a baby absorb zinc from breast milk, which would explain the protective effect of breast milk against the rare disease acrodermatitis enteropathica.

Enzymes
Some enzymes enter the milk in the milk glands via the intercellular fluid which comes from the blood capillaries in the breast. Others come from the normal breakdown of cells in the milk glands. Two enzymes, lipase (page 26) and lactoperoxidase (page 31), have been mentioned already. Others include xanthine oxidase, aldolase, alkaline and acid phosphatases, anti-trypsin (page 33), amylase and catalase. Twenty-five enzymes have so far been identified in breast milk and most are present in highest concentration soon after birth

So much for the substances we *know* to be present in milk. There are undoubtedly many others that we simply haven't yet isolated, some of which may be extremely important. After all, just because something is present in large amounts or is easy to measure doesn't necessarily mean it's especially important. Perhaps some valuable constituents of breast milk are as yet unknown. It's for this reason that manufacturers of baby milks must be fighting a losing battle.

How breast milk changes
Neither breast milk nor milk direct from a cow is of constant composition. Their make-up varies according to the length of lactation, the time of day and even within a feed itself. In the case of a cow's milk these variations affect only her calf. The bottle-fed baby drinks milk of a highly consistent composition because many cows' milk of many different types and stages is pooled for human consumption. Breast milk, on the other hand, is supplied on a 'one off' basis direct from producer to consumer and varies in composition considerably in any one woman and from one woman to another. These variations, far from being harmful, are of considerable importance as we shall now see.

Colostrum

This is the first milk made by the breast and is produced by the milk glands even before the baby is born. It is also produced for several days after birth. Colostrum is rich in protein (nine times as rich as mature milk), cells, certain amino acids, minerals (including zinc and calcium) and vitamins A, E, B_6 and B_{12} and has less fat and sugar than later milk. By the time a breastfed baby is one week old it has five times the vitamin E that a bottle-fed baby has in its body. A difference readily apparent to the mother is that her very first milk looks yellower than the milk that follows. Most important, though, is the fact that the protein fraction of colostrum contains large amounts of antibodies – the same ones that are present in later milk but many more of them. These give the newborn baby resistance to infection at a time when he would otherwise be particularly susceptible. The antibodies also coat the gut lining, which not only prevents organisms from entering the bloodsteam but also blocks the absorption of proteins which might set up allergic responses.

Bottle-fed babies in the western world don't even get cows' colostrum, let alone human colostrum, yet dairy cows' colostrum ('beestings') is considered so vital for calves that farmers save it for them or even go to the expense of buying it if necessary.

Colostrum looks thick and yellow and often leaks from the nipples during the second half of pregnancy. Soon after birth it becomes more milky and is sometimes called 'transitional milk'. Transitional milk, in turn, changes to mature milk but there is no sudden change from one to the other. There is not a fixed amount of colostrum, as many people think, so expressing it ante-natally will not reduce the total supply available to the baby. Letting the baby suck frequently and for as long as he wants in the first few days will not only give him more of the valuable colostrum but will also hasten the production of mature milk and will condition the let-down reflex to work quickly and efficiently (see page 12).

The low fat content of colostrum is advantageous to the newborn baby because he secretes little lipase of his own and would have difficulty in digesting larger amounts of fat in the first day or so.

An anti-trypsin enzyme in colostrum (also present in mature milk) helps prevent the digestion of antibodies by trypsin in the gut. Antibodies, as we've seen, are proteins and the gut's trypsin breaks down proteins under normal circumstances. To ensure that these life-saving antibodies are not destroyed, colostrum contains this special anti-trypsin enzyme.

Mature milk

This contains a fifth of the protein of colostrum and more fat and sugar. It is thinner-looking and whiter or even bluish-white. During the first year of breastfeeding the protein content of breast milk gradually falls, regardless of the mother's diet. This is compensated for by the fact that most babies are given increasing amounts of solid foods from about six months and these provide the extra protein necessary for growth. Also, don't forget that the baby is growing at its fastest in the first six months of life when the level of protein in breast milk is at its highest. The fall-off in protein is paralleled by a normal reduction in growth rate.

As we saw in the last chapter, the early part of a feed is made of the foremilk which is low in fat while the later part is the hindmilk with four to five times the amount of fat and one-and-a-half times as much protein. Some mixing occurs if the let-down operates before the baby has finished all the foremilk. This happens more in the second breast. Foremilk tends to look relatively thin and white or bluish-white, while hindmilk is thicker and creamy-white. The important thing to be learned from this is that feeds should continue until the baby is satisfied and not be stopped after an arbitrary length of time when the hindmilk may not be finished and may not even have been let down. Many hungry babies whose mothers think they are not producing enough milk are getting only the low calorie foremilk before the mother stops feeding. As a result the baby actually loses weight or fails to gain and is soon started on cows' milk supplements.

The changing composition of milk during a feed means that a baby finishes feeding at the first breast with high fat milk and then carries on at the second breast with lots of thin, watery foremilk. Babies have been seen to stop feeding at the first breast even though there is still milk there. They then go on to feed with vigour at the second breast, much to everyone's surprise. Similarly, babies often stop feeding at the second breast of their own accord even though there is plenty of milk there. This may well be because the baby has had enough of the fat-rich hindmilk. The concentration of fat in breast milk is least in the early hours of the morning.

Regression milk

As a baby takes less and less milk from the breast, the milk looks more like colostrum – thicker and yellower. Some women find they are able to express this milk from their breasts many months after they have stopped feeding their babies.

So now we've examined the complexity and specificity of breast milk, is it fair to assume that bottle-fed babies do badly? The answer is that while the vast majority of bottle-fed babies in the West thrive, more of them suffer from certain illnesses during their first year and there may be some long-term effects of drinking cows' milk in infancy which we are only now beginning to appreciate. We'll discuss this more in Chapter 4. The basic thing we've tried to get across in this chapter is that breast milk *is* different from cows' milk, even if the cows' milk is modified. It's no longer reasonable for doctors and food scientists to tell the public that breast milk is equalled by cows' milk formulae – today we know better.

Having said this, as long as there is an alternative to breast milk, there will always be some mothers who choose not to breastfeed even though they know that breast milk is best for their babies. In other countries, especially in the Third World, it would have been better for most babies had cows' milk never been available as a substitute. The vast majority of babies in these areas would fare much better on breast milk. Many Third World families don't have enough money to buy sufficient cows' milk formula to nourish their babies adequately. Also, the babies run a high risk of developing potentially serious gastroenteritis because of their parents' ignorance about how to sterilise bottle-feeding equipment or a lack of basic facilities.

Bottle-feeding, however carefully done, can only ever be a second best. Nature gives a mother the very best for her baby.

4 Best for baby?

When weighing up the pros and cons of breastfeeding, the scale-pan falls very heavily on the side of the 'pros' and indeed when writing this and the next chapter we found it difficult to find anything much to say against breastfeeding. Even many of the 'disadvantages' that would-be breastfeeders see are readily overcome if you know how.

There is an increasing body of scientific evidence to support the medical advantages enjoyed by breastfed babies. The first reports that breastfed babies might be healthier came early this century, soon after the mass introduction of bottle-feeding. A trickle of information continued over the years and has developed into an avalanche in the last fifteen years. The medical and nursing profess-ions are not always quick to take up new information, especially if it recommends sweeping changes in the management of people in hospital and the community. This is not necessarily a bad thing and protects the public from medical fads and fancies to some extent. But in the case of breastfeeding we think that if *mothers* understand the advantages to their babies of being breastfed, then pressure from them will do more than anything to change the poor standard of help and advice available to breastfeeding women in some areas.

The perfect food
In the last chapter we explained the unique composition of breast milk and how the amount and type of each foodstuff is just right for your baby. But breast milk doesn't simply provide food, as we shall now see.

Perfect for growth
Bottle-fed babies tend to put on weight faster than breastfed ones. However, optimum growth isn't a matter of putting on weight as quickly as possible, as many people think. The growth of the

human infant is a complex affair. When we compare the rates of growth of infants in developing countries with those in ours we find that their 'underprivileged' children grow less quickly than western children. As prosperity increases so do the growth rates of babies. But is it sensible to assume that babies that grow fast are what we should be aiming for?

Apparently not, if the work of a distinguished doctor in southern Africa is anything to go by. He questions whether the usual growth rate for American and British babies should be taken as normal. By their standards many millions of children are malnourished yet seem perfectly fit and well and grow up to be healthier than many western children. A hundred years ago English children reached their maximum height at the age of twenty-five; today they get there at sixteen. Among the rural Bantu in Africa today the age is twenty.

Animal experiments have shown that slower growth rates in the young make for slower ageing and this seems to be borne out in humans if we accept evidence from South Africa where in one study there were at least twenty times as many Bantu over the age of 100 as there were whites. This is well worth thinking about because it may be that by overfeeding our children we could be accelerating their growth and the onset of degenerative diseases, so decreasing their life span. It's difficult to overfeed grossly if you're solely breast-feeding yet it's the easiest thing in the world if you're using cows' milk to which you can also add cereals and sugar.

There is every reason to suppose that the proportions and types of nutrients in breast milk are perfectly geared to the optimum rate of growth of babies. It's possible that any tampering with this may produce problems.

Fewer infections

We saw in the last chapter that breast milk contains factors that protect a baby from infection by bacteria, viruses, yeasts and other organisms. This sounds good but in practical terms how important is it today when hygienic precautions for bottle-feeding are so good and the treatment of infections is so advanced?

For two thirds of the world's population, feeding babies with cows' milk formula is 'tantamount to signing a death warrant', according to the United Nations Protein Advisory Group. The risk of these babies developing infective diarrhoea is extremely high, because of the lack of adequate hygiene precautions together with the lack of anti-infective factors in cows' milk. In the western world we don't have the high infant mortality figures that we had in the earlier part of this century but many thousands of babies still suffer from gastroenteritis and respiratory infections (colds, coughs, ear infections, pneumonia, bronchitis, bronchiolitis and flu, to name but a few). An important organism causing respiratory infection is the respiratory syncitial virus. Breastfeeding has been shown to protect a baby against this organism. Some babies get other serious infections such as meningitis and septicaemia. Though we can prevent most of these babies from actually dying, no mother wants to see her baby in hospital or even suffering from repeated infections at home. *Breastfeeding will help protect your baby against these infections, especially if you breastfeed exclusively.* It is now almost certain that even one feed of bottle milk can so alter the environment within a baby's bowel (albeit temporarily) that he may pick up an infection that a wholly breastfed baby would not.

In Manchester in 1970, out of 170 babies under six months old admitted to a hospital with gastroenteritis, *only one* baby was being breastfed!

In Newcastle in 1976, among babies treated for respiratory infections, only one baby in fourteen was being breastfed, compared with one in four among healthy babies outside the hospital.

If we look further afield, we can find even more startling figures. In parts of rural China in 1973, bottle-fed babies had twice the chance of dying as had breastfed babies. In Guatemala in 1971, experienced workers reported that gastroenteritis was unknown in the breastfed but common in bottle-fed babies. And among Canadian Eskimos in 1971, middle ear infections were five times as common in the bottle-fed.

We know that today the vast majority of western mothers prepare feeds hygienically. So it must be that the many anti-infective factors in breast milk are responsible in a *positive way* for the resistance of the breastfed to infection.

Two rare diseases of babies that we'll mention here are necrotising enterocolitis – a bowel infection with a high death rate seen almost exclusively in the bottle-fed – and acrodermatitis enteropathica, a disease for which breast milk provides the only treatment (see page 32). These are rare diseases but virtually never seen in breastfed children.

Fewer allergic diseases

There are probably few subjects in child care that have stimulated so much interest and concern in recent years as has infantile eczema and it continues to be a distressing and difficult condition to treat. An American study in Chicago that followed over 20,000 babies for five years found that there were seven times as many babies with eczema in the bottle-fed group as in those completely breastfed. (Babies given some breast and some bottle milk were twice as likely to get eczema as the totally breastfed ones.) This survey also found that one in twenty babies fed on cows' milk developed eczema!

In fact, more than 30,000 babies are known to develop cows' milk allergy every year in the USA and there must be many more that simply aren't diagnosed.

This research into allergy is fascinating. It is estimated that approximately thirty-one million people (15 per cent of the population) in the US suffer from some sort of allergic disorder. It has been known for some time that eczema, asthma and hay fever are less common in children who have been breastfed. We now know that many other illnesses are caused by allergy to cows' milk protein or to other food proteins that pass through the gut wall of bottle-fed babies.

As we mentioned in the last chapter, babies begin to make their own immunoglobulin A (IgA) only after the first few weeks of life. Until they make enough, they need IgA from their mother's milk. Cows' milk IgA is no help as it is spoilt by heat treatment. IgA is important in preventing allergic diseases because it forms a protective coating over the gut lining and not only fights infection there but also stops large protein molecules (such as infective organisms or proteins from cows' milk or solid foods) leaking through the gut wall into the bloodstream.

In babies who are bottle-fed there is no protective coating of IgA until the baby makes enough of his own (probably not for three months or so). Thus food proteins can leak into the bloodstream through the gut wall and be taken to various parts of the body where, in susceptible babies, they set up an allergic response. The baby is said to be sensitised. This allergy may not produce symptoms straight away but may take a while to show itself. *A single bottle of cows' milk can sensitise a susceptible baby and so possibly cause allergic symptoms either at once, when he next takes cows' milk, or some time later.* Some allergists believe that once a young baby is sensitized to one food, sensitization to other foods is made much easier. The only way of proving whether symptoms are caused by an allergy or not is to remove what is thought to be the offending food from the baby's diet, to wait for the symptoms to disappear, and then to reintroduce the food and see whether the same symptoms recur. This has been done with cows' milk protein allergy and the case proved many times over.

Why haven't we heard about this before, we can hear you say, and does cows' milk allergy cause any other problems?

Until recently, the diagnosis of cows' milk allergy or allergy to any other food was not clinically respectable, and medical students were scarcely taught about it. Various studies have suggested that between about ½ per cent and 7 per cent of bottle-fed babies are affected by an allergy to cows' milk. Symptoms produced vary tremendously and include diarrhoea, vomiting, failure to thrive, bleeding from the gut with consequent anaemia, colic, eczema, nettle rash, runny nose, cough, wheezing and rattling of the chest, asthma and bronchiolitis.

The food protein most commonly involved is the ß-lactoglobulin in cows' milk. There is no ß-lactoglobulin in breast milk. Boys seem to be affected twice as often as girls and the symptoms seem to be more common in families with a tendency to allergic problems. A baby does not have all the various symptoms at once and they may come and go with spontaneous remissions between attacks. The child who always seems to have a cold may in fact be allergic to some particular foodstuff and the 'cold' may be an allergic condition of the lining of the nose (allergic rhinitis) and not a viral infection at all.

In a study of eczema in children it was found that among children from 'allergic' families, 50 per cent developed eczema in infancy if they were bottle-fed whereas only 8 per cent did if they were breastfed. As breastfeeding obviously gives such protection against eczema in these circumstances and as eczema can be such an unpleasant complaint, this argument alone is a strong point in favour of breastfeeding.

In a study in Lancashire 90 per cent of mothers with an allergic family history were able to breastfeed in hospital and 80 per cent were still feeding at three months. This remarkably high level of success was due to two factors. First, the doctors were very encouraging and the women had plenty of back-up help and, second, they were highly motivated because they were so convinced of the value of breastfeeding to their potentially allergic children.

It is possible for breast milk to contain traces of 'foreign' foods (such as cows' milk, egg, cereal, nuts and fish) which can cause allergic symptoms in highly susceptible babies. This helps explain why a few breastfed babies develop eczema, asthma or other allergic conditions such as colic. If a mother wants to know whether her baby's symptoms might be caused by a food she is eating getting through into her breast milk, she will need to do a trial of food avoidance (an elimination diet) and challenge. The suspect food should be removed from her diet for about a week. If the baby's symptoms improve, she can later try eating that food again to see if it really was the culprit. Cows' milk is the most obvious food to eliminate first, but remember that 'hidden' cows' milk is present in lots of foods. Only one food should be avoided at a time, otherwise no one will be any the wiser. It's interesting that some immunologists think that the traces of undigested foodstuffs from the mother's diet in her milk may be nature's way of preparing the baby's digestive and immunological systems for direct contact with food other than breast milk later. Similar preparation probably begins even earlier with the transplacental passage of foodstuffs to the unborn baby. Only occasionally is a baby so sensitive that these food traces (or 'dietary antigens') cause allergic problems.

Mothers of susceptible babies should as far as possible avoid eating large amounts of any one food at any one time, and especially cows' milk and eggs.

Other ways in which a baby can get eczema and asthma are by the inhalation of or skin contact with 'foreign' proteins.

Less coeliac disease

Coeliac disease is a condition seen in children after they begin to eat cereals and is caused by the gut's inability to handle the protein *gluten* which is present in wheat, rye, barley and oats. The gut lining is damaged by this protein so that the digestion of various foods is impaired. Such children fail to thrive and have a swollen abdomen and foul-smelling stools. Treatment consists of completely withdrawing gluten from the diet. A recent UK government report on infant feeding advised that babies should not be given cereals (or indeed any solids) before three months at the earliest in order to protect young babies from the possibility of getting coeliac disease.

It seems likely that the IgA coating of the gut lining in young breastfed babies may prevent this damage by gluten. In any case it seems wise not to give cereals at least until the baby is making enough of his own IgA after the first three months or so. In a survey in western Ireland where only 3 per cent of babies were breastfed, coeliac disease was about four times as common as in England where many more babies were breastfed.

Less ulcerative colitis and Crohn's disease

These two diseases of later life may be connected with the type of feeding in infancy and especially the early introduction of solids. In one survey it was found that people with ulcerative colitis were twice as likely as 'normal' people never to have been breastfed.

Another study showed that people with long-standing ulcerative colitis had high levels of antibodies to cows' milk protein in their blood.

More research into this aspect of these diseases is obviously needed. The difficulty with this sort of research is that few adults know exactly how they were fed as babies, so the researchers need to ask the subjects' *mothers* for details, which is a time-consuming and sometimes impossible business.

Fewer sudden infant deaths (cot deaths)

Some babies die suddenly and unexpectedly (often at around four months) with no obvious cause being found at post mortem. A viral illness is suggested in many cases. The babies may go to sleep normally and then die in their sleep. In the US sudden infant death is the leading cause of death in babies aged between one month and one year. In the UK two in every 1,000 babies die in this way – a total of 1,800 babies a year! It is not difficult to imagine the immense suffering caused to the families of these children.

Research into the association between feeding and sudden infant deaths is rather confused as many workers talk only about the method of feeding during the first few weeks of life and not that just before the time of death. What does emerge, though, is that the risk to a breastfed baby is very much less than that to a bottle-fed baby. Even if breastfeeding is only done for a short time some protection is conferred against the risk of death later. There have been isolated cases of *entirely* breastfed babies dying in this way but these seem to be rare.

No one knows why these babies die, though lots of ideas are being investigated. Some researchers have suggested that there might be a sudden overwhelming allergic response to a 'foreign' protein such as cows' milk protein. Another idea is that the baby is killed by a viral invasion with which he is completely unable to cope. Because breast milk contains no 'foreign' protein (except for occasional traces of the mother's food) and also provides resistance against many viral infections, these facts alone suggest that a good way of preventing many of these tragic deaths would be for all babies to be completely breastfed for *at least* the first three months.

Less obesity

We've become very weight conscious, especially over the last decade or so, partly because we know that fat people are more prone to heart disease, high blood pressure, diabetes, varicose veins and gallstones and also have a reduced life expectancy.

The statement that fat babies become fat adults is an oversimplification and in many cases not true. However, there is certainly an overall tendency for this to happen, especially if the rate of weight gain in early infancy is high. It has been shown that 10 to 20 per cent of fat babies will be fat when they are between five and seven years old. Of babies whose weight is over the ninetieth percentile, about 14 per cent are obese adults twenty to thirty years later. This means that most (over 80 per cent) fat babies are likely to lose their excess fat after infancy. However, half of all obese children were fat as babies. Whether or not obesity in breastfed babies should be prevented by giving them fewer and/or shorter feeds is debatable. Their fat stores act as depots in times of serious illness, so perhaps nature should be left alone. The only time when it is obviously sensible to cut down on breastfeeds is if you're in the habit of misinterpreting your baby's restlessness or cries as signs that he wants the breast when in fact he wants attention of other kinds, for example simply to be talked to or played with. It's only too easy to 'stuff' the breast in the baby's mouth and carry on talking to a friend! What is certain is that the habit of eating too much is easily implanted in a young child. While we have all seen fat breastfed babies, there is statistically more chance of a baby being fat if he is bottle-fed, as many surveys have shown. In one such study in Sheffield in 1971, 60 per cent of bottle-fed babies put on too much weight in the first year compared with only 19 per cent of breastfed babies.

One of the reasons for this is that the high mineral content of cows' milk makes babies thirsty and if their thirst is quenched by more milk, the extra calories it contains make them fat. The recent modification of cows' milk preparations, which means that their mineral content is better controlled, may reduce this danger to some extent. However, some mothers will always give their babies 'an extra scoop for the pot', especially before bedtime and this just can't happen when a baby is breastfed. Another reason is that it's easy to put some cereal powder into the bottle in a (fruitless) attempt to make the baby sleep longer. Breastfeeding mothers are much less likely to give their babies early solids.

Less heart disease
Many people are amazed at the suggestion that heart disease could possibly have anything to do with baby milk. Several research reports must make them think again.

A study of a hundred bodies of young people aged up to twenty who had died from various unrelated causes showed that abnormalities in the coronary arteries were more common in those who had been bottle-fed. Abnormality in the coronary arteries is the major problem underlying angina and heart attacks so is clearly worth worrying about. One in three middle-aged men in the western world dies of heart disease.

There are several theories as to why this should be. Some have suggested that the arterial damage in the bottle-fed is a result of the action of antibodies to cows' milk protein which are found in bottle-fed babies. More recently it has been suggested that the antibodies causing the damage are antibodies to cows' milk cream – more specifically, to the milk fat globule membrane. Others think that the different fat composition and content of cows' milk may be responsible.

The discovery that men under sixty who have heart attacks have higher than normal levels of antibodies to cows' milk protein made a lot of people sit up and rethink their ideas. It has also been found that a man who has had a heart attack has three times more chance of dying from it if he has any cows' milk antibodies in his blood at all.

Although breastfed babies *can* develop antibodies to cows' milk later in life, there is evidence that when they do their antibody levels are lower than those of people who were fed on cows' milk formula as infants.

Cows' milk protein causes the formation of antibodies in susceptible people when they drink it. These antibodies or 'immune complexes' are known to make the blood more sticky and so predispose towards clot formation. The ability to produce antibodies to cows' milk protein may well be inherited: one family in which there was a very high level of heart disease had antibody levels eight times those seen in the normal population.

Although the research is not as yet conclusive, it seems likely that some bottle-fed babies become sensitised by cows' milk protein, develop antibodies to it and so become more likely to suffer from heart attacks in later life. Even if this theory offers only a glimmer of hope, the fact remains that degenerative arterial disease is a forerunner of angina and heart attacks – diseases so serious and common in the western world that any suggestion of a causative factor should be taken very seriously.

It's important to stress that we're not suggesting that breastfeeding will completely prevent heart attacks. Heart disease is so complex and the numbers of factors involved so many that even though bottle-feeding is possibly one of the factors, it certainly isn't the only one.

Less dental decay

The breastfed baby is less likely to suffer from dental decay when he is older than the bottle-fed baby, a fact which is little known. Dental decay not only costs the nation a lot of money (only mental disease costs more) but, more important, it causes children a lot of pain and brings with it the risk of having to have false teeth. Just bear in mind that 37 per cent of all the people in the UK over the age of sixteen have no teeth of their own and you'll see how serious the problem is. There are twenty-two million people who actually have false teeth and we have seen four-year-olds with complete sets of dentures!

So why is the breastfed baby protected? We don't know for certain but there seem to be two mechanisms at work. Firstly, the fluoride level in breast milk is increased in areas with high levels of fluoride in the drinking water. It seems that cows' milk produced in fluoridated water areas doesn't show as great an increase, though the fluoride content of the milk does rise slightly compared with that from non-fluoridated areas. We know that fluoride in the right dose reduces dental decay by 50 per cent, so this is one protective factor.

However, in a non-fluoridated area, the amount of fluoride in breast and bottle milk is nearly the same but breastfed babies still have reduced decay rates in early childhood. This means that another mechanism must be at work. In one survey it was shown that children breastfed for more than three months in an area with little fluoride in the water had a 46-per-cent reduction in the incidence of dental decay compared with bottle-fed children. In practical terms this meant that the numbers of decayed, missing or filled teeth were almost twice as high in those children who had been bottle-fed.

Before you jump to the conclusion that this was obviously because of the sugar added to the babies' bottles, the research workers thought of that and managed to show that sugar was not involved in the differences seen.

The same sort of study in a different area with fluoridated water showed that children breastfed for more than three months had a 50-per-cent reduction in the incidence of dental decay compared with the bottle-fed.

Better jaw and mouth development

Many specialists report that they see fewer problems of faulty jaw and mouth development in breastfed babies. Indeed, in one survey of nearly 500 children with such problems only two had been breastfed. The underlying cause seems to be the abnormal action of the muscles of the mouth and tongue that a bottle-fed baby learns when sucking and swallowing from the bottle.

This abnormal 'swallow' can produce several types of mal-occlusion (crookedness) of the teeth, all of which take much time and patience on the part of the orthodontist, child and parents to put right. Treatment for many of these disorders often means repeated trips to the dentist over a period of years – well worth preventing if possible.

Other health factors
Multiple sclerosis
Some researchers have suggested a possible connection between bottle-feeding and the later development of multiple sclerosis. Further work is in progress at present.

Pyloric stenosis
This narrowing of the opening of the gullet into the stomach (which occasionally needs an operation to cure the symptoms) has been reported to be less common in breastfed babies.

Meconium plugs and meconium ileus
These conditions can both cause blockage of the gut which may need an operation. Each is less common and less severe in breast-fed babies because colostrum stimulates the passage of meconium.

Other developmental differences
Whilst it may seem relatively unimportant, it is interesting that two studies have shown that breastfed babies walk earlier than bottle-fed babies even after allowing for differences in weight between the two groups and excluding babies whose mothers went out to work (because they might possibly have been less stimulated to walk).

Another study of nearly 400 children using several tests showed that the highest *intelligence quotients* were obtained by children who had been breastfed for between four and nine months. Five per cent of the breastfed children had IQs of 130 or higher, while none of the bottle-fed group had. Before dismissing this survey as being a lot of nonsense, it is worth considering that it's likely that the amino acid pattern of human milk is optimal for the development of the human brain, which grows tremendously fast in the first year of life.

Though the causes of behavioural differences in later childhood are impossible to pin down with certainty, one study of seven-year-olds showed that those who had been breastfed were less fearful, less nervous, less jealous and less spiteful than their bottle-fed peers. They were also more successful at school.

Attachment to mother

Scientific proof of any increased attachment to the mother if her child is breastfed is hard to come by but a closer relationship seems likely if only because the baby has to depend on his mother alone for food. She is also likely to feed him to comfort him instead of just holding him or giving him a dummy. Studies have in fact shown that breastfed babies spend less time in their cots and more with their mothers than do bottle-fed ones. In communities where unrestricted breastfeeding is not only allowed but is actively encouraged by society, mothers don't let their babies cry even for a short time. In our western society babies are unfortunately often left to cry in their cots because 'it's not time for a feed' and 'they might be spoilt if they're picked up for a cuddle'. The baby whose mother gives him the breast for food or comfort whenever he cries would seem highly likely to grow up feeling very secure in his mother's love.

Studies have shown that the behaviour of a breastfeeding mother before, during and after feeding is also different from that of a bottle-feeding mother. The mother who breastfeeds is more likely to kiss, rock and touch her baby while the bottle-feeding mother is more likely to rub, pat and jiggle her baby and will show much more concern over 'wind'. Breastfeeding mothers also talk to their babies more than bottle-feeding mothers do.

The properly breastfed baby cries from hunger less because his needs can be immediately satisfied by warm milk. The bottle-fed baby is more likely to have to wait until his mother thinks it is time for his feed and then will have to wait again while his feed is prepared and warmed and may feel very real hunger and frustration during this time. What's more, the breastfed baby can be sure of a decent meal, even in countries where his mother is relatively short of food herself, while the bottle-fed baby in a poor family may be given a dilute feed which won't satisfy him for long. This is, unfortunately, especially likely in the Third World.

So much for all the advantages of breastfeeding for your baby. Quite a list, isn't it? We often hear advocates of bottle-feeding say, 'Yes, but look at the millions of babies who have grown up healthily on cows' milk.' Our answer is that breastfed babies are, on average, *even more* healthy and also that breastfeeding *can actually save lives*. We already know of many diseases linked with bottle-feeding and who knows how many more will be discovered in the future?

Are there any disadvantages to breastfeeding from the baby's point of view? Only a few, which can be overcome.

If a mother's diet is *grossly* deficient in protein and fat (such as may happen among the starving peoples of the world) then the baby is liable to go short as well. The answer here is not to give the baby cows' milk but to give the mother more food. The World Health Organisation recently decided that in future it would concentrate famine relief monies on food for breastfeeding mothers rather than on vast and costly supplies of powdered cows' milk for babies. Babies fed on cows' milk in famine circumstances have a much greater risk of dying than do breastfed babies, because of the enormous risk of gastroenteritis from unsterilised bottles and water. They are also highly likely to be given dilute feeds so that the mother can save some supplies of milk powder in case she can't get any or can't afford any the next day.

Another problem crops up in countries where mothers eat large amounts of polished rice which is lacking in vitamin B_1 (thiamine) and develop beri-beri. Breastfed babies can become acutely ill when fed by these mothers. The solution is for health workers to teach mothers where they are going wrong – the rice should be eaten unpolished in order to provide enough vitamin B_1.

Some strictly vegetarian mothers (vegans) have low levels of Vitamin B_{12} in their milk and so give too little of this vitamin to their babies, which then develop symptoms of deficiency. Extra vitamin B_{12} for the mothers soon puts this right.

And in this country? The only serious disadvantage is probably the frustration and hunger suffered by a baby whose mother has insufficient milk for him. But this is almost always easily overcome with help and perseverance (see Chapter 10).

5 Best for you

The biological perspective

As a species human females develop breasts (and quite large ones for their size compared with other animals) very early. In most mammals the mammary glands only develop in time to feed the young but humans, whose breasts are well developed several years before childbearing begins (even in hunter-gatherer and other traditional rural peoples), clearly have them for other purposes too. The chief among these is almost certainly as a source of sexual arousal in a species of mammal that (along with the other higher primates) is unique in wanting to and being able to copulate at any time.

Man has probably been on the face of the earth for about five million years and until 5,000 years ago he lived the life of a hunter-gatherer and ate a monkey-type vegetarian diet. It seems from such evidence as is available from historical remains and from the study of the few hunter-gatherer tribes that persist in the world today that the whole reproductive life of such people is very different from our own. Perhaps the best studied hunter-gatherers of the present day are the !Kung of Botswana and Namibia who live as our ancestors did for millions of years. The women of such a tribe start to menstruate late by western standards (at about seventeen to eighteen) and their menopause is earlier – at about thirty-eight. Their total female reproductive span is therefore only about twenty years long whereas ours is about thirty-six years (from thirteen to forty-nine). Also, because they breastfeed their young on an unrestricted basis they do not ovulate for much of their reproductive lives and so often do not menstruate for years on end. Women who live like this (as indeed all of mankind did until about 5,000 years ago when they started living in settlements based on agricultural food supplies) become fertile, menstruate a few times, have their first child, breastfeed for several years and then, as their ovulation returns as breastfeeding falls off, become pregnant again and so repeat the cycle. To such women menstruation is not a monthly event but an uncommon one which occurs as a result of their relatively few ovulatory cycles. They have perhaps six or seven children, some of whom die at birth or during the first year, and so they end up with a family of three or four children.

So the pattern overall is that hunter-gatherer women are either pregnant or breastfeeding for almost the whole of their reproductive lives. This in turn means that instead of experiencing the 400–450 menstrual cycles of the modern western woman they have only twenty to thirty in a whole lifetime.

This then was the picture for all women until a mere 5,000 years ago – a drop in the ocean in terms of evolution. Biologically we are still more akin to these hunter-gatherers than to anyone else, yet over the past 200 years of industrial life we have dramatically changed our way of life to one in which women now start menstruating earlier and earlier and have regular monthly menstrual cycles with their accompanying surges of hormones on hundreds of occasions until the menopause intervenes at about the age of fifty. Changes have been, of course, occuring over thousands of years but it seems that our very recent change in life-style has accelerated things considerably.

Just what all this does to modern women we don't yet know but we can be sure that her body wasn't made to cope with such abnormal patterns. Our females' reproductive systems have evolved to behave in one way yet today's way of life forces them to behave in quite another.

But, we can hear you say, all these hunter-gatherers must have a child every three or four years, spaced only by their breastfeeding contraception. I don't want a child every three years, so what relevance has all this for me? Certainly this is a valid objection. Today in the West, when the vast majority of children survive, being pregnant or breastfeeding for much of the time, as the hunter-gatherer women are, would result in families larger than society would consider acceptable.

What has all this to do with a book on breastfeeding? Quite simply the breast is an integral part of a woman's reproductive system. Her breasts are linked into the same hormonal systems that operate during orgasm, childbirth, breastfeeding and her menstrual cycle – in other words, during her whole reproductive life.

There is absolutely no doubt that breast cancer (now the commonest cancer killer in women) has become more common over the last two hundred years and that benign (non-cancerous) conditions of the breast are enormously common. It has been estimated that one in twenty women in the West today will die of breast cancer and that one in four will suffer from some sort of breast condition.

Why should this be? Why should women's breasts be so prone to disease? The answer probably lies in the extraordinary way that we treat them – a way which is so recent in evolutionary terms that our bodies haven't had a chance to adapt to it. Breastfeeding is still the single most important method of contraception around the world yet few women in the so-called 'enlightened' West realise it. By breastfeeding so little or even not at all we rob the breasts of one of their main functions and the high incidence of breast disorders may be the price we are paying. And it's not only the breast that's suffering. Endometrial cancer (cancer of the lining of the uterus) is clearly linked to the incidence of breast cancer, so perhaps the 450 menstrual periods today's modern western woman experiences in her lifetime are playing havoc with her uterus too. After all, each month, if she is ovulating, a woman's body gets ready for a pregnancy. Her breasts, uterus and ovaries undergo profound physiological and anatomical changes. Many of these changes involve the growth of new cells and the stimulation of cellular RNA. It's but a short step in cellular terms from the repeated normal overgrowth of cells to their abnormal overgrowth in the form of a cancer. The whole system is keyed up ready for the fertilisation of the egg each month. In our modern world, however, an egg gets fertilised only once or twice in about 450 cycles (compared with seven or eight times in around thirty cycles in the hunter-gatherer women) – all the other cycles are 'wasted' in biological terms. This would be no great tragedy if it weren't for the fact that these profound bodily changes are repeatedly being frustrated year after year and that clearly they weren't meant to be. This may be why modern woman has such an enormous amount of reproductive organ illness. Cancer of the breast and endometrium are alarmingly common and one in five women in the UK ends up having her uterus removed. Few babies are breastfed for long, robbing them of the provable advantages of breastfeeding that go way beyond simple nutrition – can this be right?

Without being unnecessarily doom-laden we are faced with some pretty horrifying facts and our modern life seems to be geared to perpetuating the horrors rather than to alleviating them.

What can be done then to try to redress the balance, at least a little?

There's very little we can do in 1983 to make girls start menstruating later. It has been found that the age at first menstruation is linked to the nutritional status of a community so perhaps by stopping *over-nourishing* our children we could delay puberty, if only for a few years.

Once a girl starts menstruating she should, from a biological point of view, start having children within a very few years. One of the greatest proven preventives against breast cancer, for example, is having a first baby young (under twenty). The female reproductive system wasn't designed to function for a decade or more before its first baby and if we continue to insist that it does so we'll continue to have problems. This at first sight entails a complete change in society which is unlikely to come about rapidly, if at all. However, the pharmaceutical companies are looking for an answer. They are working on synthetically produced hormones that mimic those produced by the pituitary gland of the woman who is constantly pregnant or breastfeeding. Work is under way to isolate and prepare such substances. When such a compound exists a girl could keep her hormone profile in such a state that she would not ovulate. Once she was rendered anovulatory in this way she would then behave biologically like the !Kung and her hunter-gatherer ancestors and would almost certainly have fewer breast and other reproductive ailments and diseases. Anovulation isn't the whole answer because it is possible that the hormones of pregnancy and breastfeeding may be protective too.

Of course, the ideal answer would be for women to go back to a more natural pattern of reproduction but this is unlikely to occur in the foreseeable future unless society changes dramatically for some reason. Few societies in the world today can afford the increase in population that would go with a return to such a reproductive life-style.

Once a woman starts having babies her whole reproductive system *can* be influenced, if only for a few years, by breastfeeding on an unrestricted basis. From a nutritional point of view there is very little point in breastfeeding much beyond eight months or so in the western world but from the *woman's* point of view there is every reason for carrying on with frequent feeds, even if the child is getting much of his nourishment from other foods. With frequent nipple stimulation the mother's hormone levels usually remain in a condition which prevents ovulation for many months. This not only acts as a natural contraceptive but also prevents the monthly changes that we have seen can be so harmful when repeated year after year.

In this way the woman could enjoy a year or more of post-baby anovulation and this, together with nine months of pregnancy, gives her two years or so per baby of more biologically normal reproductive behaviour. Even two children per woman would then give four years of protection and it's possible that the benefits in biological terms increase with the more children she has, provided they are all breastfed for a long time.

The current situation over women's reproductive ills is hardly ideal but perhaps we shall see a return to more biological mothering, earlier childbearing and, who knows, even a return to a more stable family life as a result. We live in a world geared to women behaving totally abnormally in biological terms and we are probably paying the price in many ways – not the least in breast disease.

Advantages to you
Satisfaction
The mother who breastfeeds her baby successfully for as long as she and the baby want is likely to get a lot of satisfaction even if she doesn't know about all the very real advantages to the baby. Many mothers say that they felt a tremendous sense of loss when they gave their baby his last breastfeed. Perhaps this is partly because a breastfed baby is even more dependent upon his mother for his food than is a bottle-fed one, and the majority of mothers enjoy this feeling of being needed. Whilst on the subject of satisfaction it is interesting that in a survey of recently delivered mothers, those who were 'greatly pleased' with their babies were much more successful at breastfeeding than those who were 'indifferent'.

Enjoyment
One of the advantages that people often forget to mention is that overall most mothers find breastfeeding enjoyable. There's something

very special about the pleasure of having a baby at your breast staring up into your eyes and perhaps stopping sucking every now and then when he breaks into a smile. Being able to comfort your baby easily and quickly at any time and anywhere is another bonus. Bottle-feeding mothers never have the pleasure of lying down by their baby as they feed. You can cuddle into your breastfeeding baby as you lie by him at night (or during the day if you rest together) and may even doze off as he feeds.

Fulfilment

Another feeling often expressed is that breastfeeding is one of the things that only a woman can do – like giving birth. In today's world of sexual equality and unisex this feminine fulfilment is valued not only by the naturally maternal but also by the erstwhile career woman who sees her enjoyment of breastfeeding as representing the female part of her character. This oneness that many breastfeeding women feel with their babies is often quoted as the major advantage to breastfeeding mothers. Certainly they often seem to be more at ease with their babies.

Getting your figure back

Three months after her baby is born the breastfeeding mother is more likely to be losing weight without dieting than the mother who is bottle-feeding. Breastfeeding uses up some of the fat stores accumulated during pregnancy and so naturally helps a woman get back to her pre-pregnancy shape and weight provided that she is not overeating. If the shape of the breasts is altered at all, it will probably be because of the pregnancy and not the breastfeeding. Breasts tend to return to their normal shape and size about six months after weaning. Various women report that their breasts are either smaller, larger or droopier after breastfeeding but there is no general trend.

Convenience

A big practical point in favour of breastfeeding is that it really is more convenient. More convenient not only at home, where there are no bottles and teats to wash and sterilise and no feeds to prepare, but also when you go out as there is no equipment to get ready and take with you. Holidays become a much more practical proposition and car rides with the baby can actually be pleasant. Not for you the cooling of a bottle of hot milk by holding it out of the car window at great speed! And no spilt milk powder over the car seats.

The breastfeeding mother needs only her baby and a clean nappy to go anywhere and it takes only a little ingenuity and forethought to be able to breastfeed anywhere without embarrassment to you or anyone else.

Another thing that only a mother who has both breastfed and bottle-fed at different times will know is that it's nearly always possible to comfort an infant by giving him the breast, even if he's not particularly hungry. Bottle-fed babies often don't seem to be comforted by sucking on a bottle of water or a dummy – unless you're lucky. This means that a household with a breastfed baby is quieter and happier all round than one with a bottle-fed baby, provided you as his mother are willing to let him be comforted by suckling him whenever he cries.

Cost

The question of the relative cost of bottle-feeding as against breast-feeding is not really of very great importance in western countries. A few pennies here or there will not influence the average woman either way.

To the cost of dried milk powder needs to be added the cost of bottles, teats, sterilising tablets or gas or electricity to boil the equipment, when working out the cost of bottle-feeding. A bottle-feeding mother will need several bottles and teats over the total period and the cost of these soon adds up.

A breastfeeding mother needs to consider the cost of the extra food she should be eating each day in order to produce enough milk. Experts think that she needs to eat enough extra food to provide her with 300 to 500 calories a day over and above her normal intake. The baby will take more from her than this amount but the difference is made up by the calories obtained from the fat stores she laid down during pregnancy. This is why a breastfeeding mother will carry on losing weight (unless she eats too much) until she stops breastfeeding.

Obviously the cost of extra food will depend entirely on what sort of food the breastfeeding mother chooses to eat – if she takes her extra calories as best steak it'll work out far more expensive than if she takes them as sandwiches. If she just eats a little more of everything than she normally eats, then the cost of the extra food is lower than the cost of bottle-feeding a baby. This is especially important in the developing countries where many mothers literally cannot afford to buy enough cows' milk powder for their babies but can just about afford to buy some extra food for themselves.

Birth control

The contraceptive effect of breastfeeding was dismissed as an old wives' tale until very recently. This is doubly amazing as it is the only contraceptive known to the majority of the world's women. It is quite true that a woman is less likely to conceive while breastfeeding even if she uses no other form of contraception but what is not so often realised is that it *is* possible for her to conceive while still breastfeeding. The amount of protection depends upon whether the baby relies solely on breast milk, on the length of time between feeds, and on whether the baby is allowed to feed for comfort after or between feeds.

Why should conception be less likely? The answer seems to be that the high levels of the hormone prolactin in the breastfeeding mother inhibit the response of her ovaries to the pituitary gland's follicle-stimulating hormone. Ovulation therefore doesn't occur and pregnancy can't happen.

However, prolactin levels naturally fall throughout lactation, even in a fully breastfeeding mother, so there comes a time when they are no longer high enough to prevent ovulation. In *fully* breastfeeding women this doesn't happen until around the tenth week at the earliest but even then *only one woman in twenty* will ovulate before the eighteenth week after childbirth.

In women who don't breastfeed at all, ovulation occurs *on average* eight to ten weeks after the birth of their babies; this means that one in two will be at risk of becoming pregnant before her baby is eight to ten weeks old unless she uses some other form of contraception.

The partially breastfeeding mother will not ovulate for longer than the average bottle-feeding mother but will ovulate before.

It is not safe to wait for your first period before you start using contraception because 5 per cent of women ovulate before their first period. Usually, though, the first few menstrual cycles after childbirth are anovular.

Many studies in far-flung parts of the world suggest that the birth controlling effect of breastfeeding is more powerful there than in the western world. The interval between babies is around two to three years for many women in developing countries. Breastfeeding mothers in these countries are often undernourished and this can cause a delay in ovulation. In some cultures there are tribal taboos on sexual intercourse with lactating women. However, the main reason behind their prolonged lactation contraception is that many of these women are far more likely than we are to practise completely *unrestricted* breastfeeding. The sort of full breastfeeding most often seen in the western world is based on the baby having five or six feeds a day (which is really only token breastfeeding) whereas babies in the rest of the world are put to the breast many more times than this. When there are long periods between suckling, which there are with only five or six feeds a day, the high prolactin levels in the blood aren't kept up. It is thought that the low levels of prolactin occurring in these long intervals between feeds allow ovulation to occur.

Similarly, when the baby is given solids or supplementary bottle-feeds he gradually relies less and less on breast milk for his nourishment and the decreased suckling soon lowers prolactin levels and allows ovulation to occur.

It seems sensible for the western woman not to *rely* on breast-feeding as a method of contraception, even if she feeds frequently, though she need not worry about using any other method for the first ten weeks if she's *fully breastfeeding* her baby on an unrestricted basis in the natural way. In contrast, the bottle-feeding mother is well advised to use some form of birth control as soon as she starts having intercourse again.

Some couples may not feel strongly about planning the intervals between their children's births exactly. If this is the case, then the prolonged contraceptive effect of *unrestricted* breastfeeding is a good method of birth control for them. In order to suppress the return of ovulation, fairly constant levels of prolactin must be maintained throughout the day and night. To do this, the baby must be put to the breast often. A long gap between episodes of suckling, as can happen if the baby sleeps a long time at night, if his mother leaves him for a long period during the day, if he uses a dummy for his comfort suckling or if he is unwell and doesn't want the breast, can so lower the prolactin levels that ovulation may occur. The *average* length of time before the return of periods in a mother who fully breastfeeds her baby on an unrestricted basis for six to eight months, then introduces solids but continues to give the breast often for drinks and for comfort, is *over fourteen months*! This goes for any mother, whatever her nationality. Couples using only lactation contraception from this sort of breastfeeding can expect an average gap between babies of around two to three years, depending on how soon ovulation returns and on their level of fertility.

Breast cancer

It has long been thought that breastfeeding protects a woman from the eventual likelihood of getting cancer of the breast and it is a fact that in those areas of the world where women spend many years of their lives breastfeeding in an unrestricted way, breast cancer is very rare indeed. But this doesn't necessarily mean that it's the breastfeeding that's protecting them and there's no evidence that such a mechanism works in western women with their 'token' breastfeeding. We still don't know what does cause this cancer – the commonest cancer in women – but there's certainly *no* evidence that breastfeeding is a contributory cause of breast cancer.

Some possible disadvantages of breastfeeding

If there are so many good reasons why breastfeeding is better for mothers, why do so many women decide not to do it at all? It would be foolish to pretend that there were no drawbacks – but they're mostly easily overcome, as we'll see.

Embarrassment

Breasts in our society have become equated with sex and women who choose to breastfeed and thus reveal their breasts are thought by many to be immodest. At the beginning of the century no one turned a hair at the sight of a woman feeding her baby in public. Now breastfeeding must be done with more than a passing thought for modesty or else the mother runs the risk of people turning to stare. This fear of embarrassment is a great off-putter to many women who may be embarrassed not only at the thought of feeding in front of complete strangers but also in front of relatives – even their husbands and children.

Because some people are embarrassed at seeing a baby at the breast, most breastfeeding mothers choose to be as discreet as possible in public. Certainly a woman doesn't have to expose her breast in order to breastfeed. If she does, a little practice in front of a mirror will make feeding in public more acceptable.

The swing back to breastfeeding in the early 1970s started with the better educated, freer thinking mothers who realised that feeding their babies offered advantages both to them and to their babies which far outweighed any feelings of embarrassment they might have had. As more and more women breastfeed, feeding in public is becoming gradually more acceptable. But until TV and other areas of the media start showing mothers feeding, the move towards acceptability will be slow.

You'll be tied

A more practical drawback to breastfeeding in our society is that it can be inconvenient because it ties the mother to her child. If she is to breastfeed successfully and fully for at least three to six months, then she'll need to be with her baby almost constantly during that time. Some mothers learn the knack of expressing enough milk into a bottle for someone else to give the baby while they go out and others give their babies the occasional bottle of cows' milk formula. Neither of these is ideal, however, unless there is no alternative, partly because until about three months some babies are still vulnerable to the effects of cows' milk protein and also because babies of this age are often unhappy to be separated from their mothers.

In the first few weeks, outings may have to be limited because the baby won't go long between feeds but even this can be overcome if you feed in the car, on a park bench or in a café where the staff are sympathetic. Discreet breastfeeds are often unnoticeable.

In some areas local NCT or LLL groups have made up lists of shops and other places where a mother may breastfeed. If no such list is available, why not consider compiling one and perhaps send it to the local paper or baby clinic.

Rather than worry about never being able to leave the baby, it's much more helpful to adopt a positive attitude and to decide to enjoy taking the baby with you everywhere you go. There are very few places that you can't go with a baby, especially a very young baby who is eminently transportable. Even the mother who has been brought up to believe that she should separate herself from her baby as much and as often as possible can change her attitude and learn to think of her baby as an extension of herself for at least a few months. The thing that young babies most like is to be with their mothers, and once you realise this you won't keep trying to leave your baby behind.

It'll hurt

Many women who have never breastfed imagine that it'll be painful and so never try.

It is true that many women who breastfeed occasionally have sore nipples and a few have other painful breast conditions. Painful nipples are only temporary and to some extent avoidable and the majority of the other painful conditions are also mostly avoidable. In a study in Blackburn nearly one woman in six who stopped breastfeeding did so because her nipples were sore. We now know that they stopped unnecessarily – their nipple soreness would have gone spontaneously if they had been helped to carry on feeding.

You can't see how much he's getting

We live in a society that measures everything, and anything that can't be measured is often regarded with suspicion. A midwife once asked us why nature didn't provide women with transparent breasts. Our answer was, why didn't bottle manufacturers make bottles in opaque material (it wouldn't have discouraged breast-feeding mothers so much)?

We've been brainwashed into thinking that it's important to know exactly how much milk the baby has taken but of course it very rarely is important, especially if the baby is healthy and thriving – which he will be if breastfeeding is properly managed. No two babies are alike and so each baby will want different amounts at different times of the day. Properly managed breastfeeding is a perfectly balanced demand and supply system.

If ever you fall into the trap of test weighing your breastfed baby to find out how much he's getting, remember that breastfed babies thrive on smaller volumes of breast milk than you would expect from comparing how much cows' milk formula bottle-fed babies take. This is partly because breast milk is perfectly digested, whereas there is so much waste with cows' milk formula that the baby needs to drink more of it to get enough nourishment.

It's unfashionable

To a certain extent, humans have a herd instinct and like to copy each other's behaviour. In maternity wards it has often been noticed by the staff that if one mother is breastfeeding successfully, newly-delivered mothers are likely to copy her. If she fails, other mothers are likely to stop breastfeeding too!

When bottle-feeding first became fashionable only the relatively wealthy could afford to buy milk powder and bottles but gradually the habit spread through all the social groups until today, when low-earning families are those most likely to contain a bottle-fed baby. The fashion is now swinging back to breastfeeding, with the middle classes leading the way.

In many hospitals now the majority of women breastfeed at least for a time but once back at home breastfeeding rates fall off very quickly.

Bottle-feeding a baby with cows' milk formula has become the normal, accepted way of behaving in the West. Most breastfed babies are soon weaned on to a bottle, though there is no need for this to happen.

You'll feel un-sexy

Some women imagine that breastfeeding will make them less sexy in their own eyes and in those of their husbands. The cult of the breast as a sex object has undoubtedly helped speed the decline of breast-feeding. The up-pointed, conical breast of the 1950s and 1960s seemed to be there solely to attract men. Certainly very few babies ever got a look in! Perhaps the recent trend towards more natural living with many young women doing without tight bras and make-up and relying more on their inborn femininity to attract men will also allow their breasts to perform their more natural function.

Disgust

A few women have a very real feeling of disgust at the idea of breastfeeding. Mothers who feel this way refuse to breastfeed at all or else give up after a day or two because to them it seems too animal-like. It's unlikely that anything will make them change their minds but one good way to help stop girls from growing up with such deep-rooted feelings is to introduce lessons mentioning breast-feeding along with other aspects of child rearing at school. Some education authorities already encourage such lessons as part of the school curriculum and in mixed schools there is the added advantage that boys can discuss the subject too. In one area of London local health educators take a nursing mother with them to these classes.

You might fail

We're convinced that the biggest disadvantage breastfeeding has in the western world is that the mother fears she'll fail and, as a result, often does. This can produce long-lasting psychological effects including a very deep sense of disappointment. So great can this feeling of failure be that many doctors and nurses have refused to tell mothers just how important it is to breastfeed their babies, for fear of their being unable to do so. This is a tragic situation not only because many mothers and babies are now not even trying but also because babies are being done out of their natural food and mothers out of their natural right – all for nothing.

The situation for many mothers today is that they feed their babies ten minutes a side every four hours or so during the day and once or not at all at night, because that is what they've been told to do. With this 'token' breastfeeding they soon find that their milk supply is dwindling – not surprisingly, because their breasts are not getting enough stimulation (see Chapter 10). Over the next few weeks they become more and more miserable as they realise their babies are not getting enough to eat and eventually they go out and buy a bottle.

There is no reason why nearly every mother should not breast-feed for as long as she wants to *provided* she understands how to make enough milk and has enough help.

A survey of expectant mothers in the UK in 1980 brought out some interesting ideas underlying their choice of feeding method.

Reasons given by mothers of first babies for choosing to breastfeed

	%
Breastfeeding is best for the baby	87
Breastfeeding is more convenient	38
Breastfeeding is natural	26
Closer bond between mother and baby	24
Breastfeeding is cheaper	22
Breastfeeding is best for mother	8
Can't overfeed the baby	3
Influenced by friends or relatives	2
Influenced by medical personnel	2
Don't know/no particular reason	1
Other reasons	1

(Percentages do not add up to 100 as some mothers gave more than one reason)

Reasons given by mothers of first babies for choosing to bottle-feed

	%
Other people can feed baby with bottle	43
Did not like idea of breastfeeding	28
Would be embarrassed to breastfeed	18
You can see how much the baby has had	18
No particular reason	10
Other reasons	6
Expecting to return to work soon	5
Persuaded by other people	3
Medical reasons for not breastfeeding	2

(Percentages do not add up to 100 as some mothers gave more than one reason.)

From *Infant Feeding*, 1980, HMSO SS1144.

The fascinating thing that emerges from these tables is that the mothers who chose to bottle-feed all gave as their reasons points against breastfeeding, not points *for* bottle-feeding. In contrast, the mothers who had decided to breastfeed were positively for breastfeeding and not for it simply because they were against bottle-feeding. Thorough discussion of the imagined disadvantages of breastfeeding in ante-natal classes, preferably with the help of a mother who is breastfeeding successfully, might go a long way to help some of these 'negative' mothers choose breastfeeding instead. Also, as the breastfeeders give the reason that breastfeeding is best for the baby as their number one choice, this must obviously be aired well and not hushed up for the sake of allaying guilt on the part of those who don't want to or really can't breastfeed.

In summary, while breastfeeding brings many advantages to mothers, it seems likely that most mothers will decide to breastfeed because of the many real advantages to their babies.

6 Preparation and pregnancy

Looking after yourself

We're going to talk here about the things you can do during pregnancy to prepare for breastfeeding your baby.

Looking after yourself is important not only for your own sake but for your family's as well. You'll be spending a large part of a year carrying, nourishing and protecting your baby and this is a long time by any standards. It's a good idea to take care to eat sensibly to maintain your health, to prepare your body for breastfeeding and to provide enough food for your developing baby. It is also sensible to get as much informed ante-natal advice as you can, to talk to your husband about your decision to breastfeed, to get in touch with people who may help you with breastfeeding should you run into any problems and generally to prepare yourself and your household so that you have as few external problems as possible when you have your new baby.

Choosing your place of birth

One of the first things you'll have to do once you know you are pregnant is book into a hospital for your delivery (unless you are going to have a home confinement). Take care when choosing where to have your baby – that is if there is a choice of hospitals in your area – because some hospitals are very much more helpful than others when it comes to breastfeeding.

If your doctor is not sure which hospital is best, ask other mothers if they were helped with breastfeeding in hospital and what sort of advice they had. If only a few mothers you talk to were completely breastfeeding on discharge from your nearest hospital, then go on inquiring until you hear of a hospital where they really do help. Even if this hospital is rather a long way from where you live, it's worth the effort of booking in there if you want to breastfeed. Even the keenest person can be discouraged if the hospital allows only schedule feeding, because that gets the establishment of successful breastfeeding off to such a bad start.

Another thing to look for is whether the hospital allows or, even better, encourages rooming-in – the practice of having the baby with the mother all the time. This system makes breastfeeding much easier and more likely to succeed.

Some hospitals have exceedingly high rates of Caesarean section, induction, painkiller use and episiotomy. Though such obstetric intervention is sometimes essential, it is wise to choose a hospital in which the majority of women are encouraged to give birth naturally, partly because breastfeeding is provably easier after a straightforward birth. More and more obstetricians are now becoming interested in helping women give birth in an upright position, rather than lying flat, as this not only speeds up the labour but also makes the contractions less arduous and increases the baby's oxygen supply. Because both mother and baby are more likely to feel well after such a birth, breastfeeding is more likely to be successful.

At your first visit you'll be asked how long you want to stay in after you have had your baby. Times vary throughout the country and some hospitals like you to stay for longer with a first baby. If you can arrange adequate help at home, you'll almost certainly get more rest at home and you'll also be able to have your baby with you all the time so that you can feed him on an unrestricted basis by day and night. Mothers who opt for a 48-hour discharge are more likely to breastfeed successfully, provided they are given enough help. This is scarcely surprising as these mothers are soon back in their own environment where they can relax. Hospital, after all, is a strange place for most of us and does little to encourage the establishment of the let-down. One American woman logged the number of intruders into her private room each day: it came to between fifty and seventy. Some chance of relaxed mothering!

Involving your husband

At some time during your pregnancy you should discuss with your husband what breastfeeding is going to mean to him. Tell him what you have learnt about the advantages of breastfeeding, give him this book to read, and take him to the fathers' night at your ante-natal class where his doubts and queries can be discussed.

He'll probably be only too pleased to fit in with the baby once he understands how important breastfeeding is. Discuss how he is going to get home after work if you usually pick him up but happen to be feeding at the time; talk about having supper at a flexible time instead of always on the dot at seven p.m.; and tell him it'll mean more sleep for you both if you have the baby sleeping with you or next to your bed so that you can feed easily during the night.

Some women choose to bottle-feed so that their husbands can sometimes enjoy giving the baby a bottle of milk. It's not natural, though, for a man to give a baby milk, so no mother should feel guilty of depriving her husband of this experience! He can enjoy cuddling the baby as much as he likes after a breastfeed.

Sources of information

Try to find out as much as possible about breastfeeding before you actually do it. Even if you have breastfed before – successfully – read about it. You'll find that later there'll be no time for reading and you may be unhappy about the things other people tell you. If you understand how breastfeeding works yourself, you'll be much more confident. Remember that all babies are different and the way they feed is totally different too. If you're thoroughly prepared for anything then you'll be more likely to manage.

Your ante-natal clinic's ante-natal classes will be valuable and with any luck there'll be a session devoted to baby feeding, a large part of which should be about breastfeeding. Try to talk to other mothers there who want to breastfeed – you may like to meet again for mutual support when you've had your babies.

A study in the UK in 1980 showed that of the mothers expecting first babies who went to ante-natal classes, 84 per cent reported that they had been told something about breastfeeding. A study in 1975 showed that when talks or discussions on infant feeding were included, only two thirds of the mothers thought that the person running the class had been in favour of breastfeeding. These mothers were more likely to plan to breastfeed than those mothers who thought no preference had been expressed. It's obvious from this that people running classes should not only include a talk about infant feeding but should also encourage breastfeeding.

You may meet your health visitor at the ante-natal class at the local clinic or surgery. She's the person who is supposed to give you advice on breastfeeding and may well be invaluable when you have your baby back home. Try to find out from other mothers if she does in fact give good, practical help. If she has the reputation for advising complementary feeds at the drop of a hat, then steer clear of her when your baby is born and go if possible to another health visitor who is more knowledgeable and supportive.

Another source of instruction is provided by the National Child-birth Trust which organises ante-natal classes throughout the country. A talk by one of their breastfeeding counsellors is included at some stage in the course and she will give you her telephone number so that you can contact her if you run into difficulties when breastfeeding. Breastfeeding counsellors are usually mothers who have had some training in counselling for breastfeeding problems. They have one advantage over many health professionals in that they have almost without exception fed babies themselves and have personal experience of some of the difficulties involved. Your counsellor will be available to talk to you over the phone at any time and will discuss things on a mother-to-mother basis. Some NCT branches arrange post-natal meetings and support groups, which are invaluable to the mother who might otherwise feel out on a limb with her new baby.

Useful discussion groups are arranged by La Leche League, a worldwide organisation of mothers who are breastfeeding or have breastfed their babies and want to help each other and anyone else with problems that may arise with breastfeeding. Anyone interested in breastfeeding is welcome to attend their meetings. The leader of your group will give you her telephone number so that you can contact her if you run into difficulties when breastfeeding. League leaders are also mothers who have learnt how to counsel mothers with breastfeeding problems. They have one advantage over many professionals in that they have all fed babies themselves. Your leader will discuss things on a mother-to-mother basis.

Bras and other clothing

From about the fifth month, or even before, your breasts will be getting larger and you'll need new bras as your breasts change over the months.

Some women manage to carry on using ordinary bras when breastfeeding, undoing them or pulling them up or down in order to feed – in fact only 40 per cent of breastfeeding women buy a special bra. Using ordinary bras can create problems as it can be difficult to do up a back-fastening bra in a hurry if a doorbell goes when you're feeding. If you simply pull the cup up or down, you'll never actually undo the bra at all, which makes things very easy. Be careful to avoid pressure under your breast from the pulled-down cup, as this can lead to a blocked duct.

It's best not to wear a bra at all when breastfeeding if you have fairly small breasts that don't need support. Some women wear a special nursing bra which opens at the front. There are two main types: one has a flap in each cup which opens to reveal the nipple and areola; the other has cups which undo completely at the centre, independently of each other. (Beware of the sort of bra that undoes completely in the middle as when undone the two halves can spring apart and be difficult to do up again.) The centre-opening bra given good support but takes time to hook (unless fastened with zips or Velcro). The flap cup bra is easy to use but unless well fitted can obstruct milk ducts by pressure from the outer circle of material left when the flap is undone. The National Childbirth Trust sells a cotton maternity and nursing bra which is available in many different sizes. It is front-opening and does up with laces at the back to allow for change in size during pregnancy and lactation. If you want a pretty nursing bra, many firms make them and they're well worth considering. Neither you nor your husband is going to feel very sexy with you in the average 'sensible' bra that many people suggest.

You will need several bras as they'll need frequent washing, especially early on when you're bound to leak. Some people find cotton more pleasant than nylon because it 'breathes' more. It's important to have the bra fitted well as it should not squash the breasts or nipples and it should also provide good support for your breasts. You may want to wear a bra at night because without one you may leak milk over the sheets in the early days. Also, because your breasts are heavier they may feel more comfortable when supported at night. However, going without a bra at night does mean that nipple soreness is less likely as the air can get to the nipples, and a terry nappy placed loosely over your breasts in bed will soak up leaks. It's much easier to put your baby to the breast at night if you're not wearing a bra!

You'll need to tuck pads of material or paper nursing pads into your bra to soak up any leaking milk. You can buy paper nursing pads (some cone-shaped) at chemists and babycare shops. Don't use paper tissues or cotton wool because these dry on to the nipples and can be difficult to remove. Some women use a square of soft material such as part of an old nappy or cut up pieces of a nappy roll. Avoid plastic-backed pads as they can prevent air from getting to the nipples and so make the skin wet and soggy.

To get back to your pregnancy, it's probably sensible to wear a good everyday bra in bed for the last three months or so. This will give your breasts the support they need to help ensure they don't get overstretched by their increased weight. After all, if you're worried about losing your figure after having children, now is the time to start caring. Maternity bras sold as sleep bras are usually too insubstantial to provide much support.

Good clothes to buy for breastfeeding include blouses, jumpers, T-shirts and anything that will pull up from the waist or do up in front. When it actually comes to feeding a good tip for discreet feeding is pull up your blouse to feed rather than undo any buttons. Some women alter their existing clothes to make them more suitable. Make sure you have several changes of clothes because nothing is more depressing than being in the same things day after day. There are lots of pretty nighties which undo in front.

Anything new you buy should be easily washable because, apart from your milk leaking, your baby may regurgitate small amounts of milk over you and dry cleaning bills can mount up very quickly with a new baby in the house.

Furniture and baby equipment

You will probably want to have the baby near you all day so you can hear him as soon as he cries. In this case you'll need either a pram, a lightweight crib, a cot on wheels or a carrycot to use downstairs. Similarly, if you want to have the baby by your bed at night for easy feeding, it's a good idea to have a readily movable cot to pull over to the bed. Babies will, of course, sleep anywhere if they are tired, warm and have a full tummy. In the early days, before they are old enough to roll, they can be put to sleep on a sofa or easy chair. The problem with this practice is that the baby may sick up some milk on to the chair covering, which may then be difficult to clean; someone may accidentally sit on him if they don't know he's there; a pet animal is more likely to interfere with him; and one day he will roll off for the first time. Some sort of cot is safer for the times when he isn't sleeping in your arms.

Some baby books talk about buying a special nursing chair and you may think it sounds like a waste of money. However, a comfortable place to feed the baby is a very real help, as it's all too easy to end up after a feed with aching shoulders and arms if you have not been as relaxed as you should be. The chair needs to be low so that your lap is flat to support the baby and it is more comfortable if your elbows are supported by cushions at the right height. Try experimenting with your existing furniture before you have the baby. A rocking chair is often pleasant for both mother and baby. Many mothers find it most comfortable to feed their babies while sitting on a sofa or bed with their feet up. Lying down to feed is the most relaxing of all!

Shopping and housework
Store as much in the way of food as you can before you have your baby. Stock up with tinned and dried food and if you have a freezer fill it if you can with prepared meals so that you and your husband can rustle up something quickly if necessary when you feel too tired to cook in the early days. Try to include as much fresh food as possible in your diet.

If you can afford it, buy stores of things like detergent, disposable nappies, terry nappy sterilising solution and ordinary household goods. When you're breastfeeding, shopping can be a problem at first as the baby may want feeding so often that there isn't much time to go out to do a large shop. You might like to find out whether any local shops deliver, though this seems to be a dying service these days. If you're lucky, your husband may volunteer to go late-night shopping sometimes, or a relative or neighbour may shop for you. This will only be for a few weeks while the baby is really small and feeding very often.

One of the great revelations to a first-time mother is the amount of laundry one small baby can generate. It's worth preparing for this well in advance. If you don't have a washing machine already see if you can possibly afford one now – it'll make all the difference to coping with terry nappies especially. If you haven't got a machine think about using a laundry for sheets and other big things for the first few weeks you're at home. This is especially important if you come home at forty-eight hours because you may soil bed clothing in the first few days.

If the chore of washing nappies without a machine is going to tire you in the early days, treat yourself to a few boxes of disposable ones. You may find they're too expensive to use after the first week or two but it'll give you a nice easy start while your milk is getting established.

Organising help at home
When you have your new baby back home, you'll need to take things slowly and easily for a few weeks and this will be much easier if you have someone to help you in the house. This is even more helpful with a second or third baby because there's more work with a family of this size. If you haven't any willing relatives nearby, you might like to arrange for paid domestic help to come in daily, though this is rather a luxury. Many husbands take a week or two off work to help out, especially if there are other children. Whatever happens, if you're going to breastfeed successfully, you'll need time to do it, especially at first when the baby will need feeding often, so don't put yourself in the role of superwoman.

Nipple and breast care
The advice given routinely to expectant mothers about how to care for their breasts and nipples has done a lot to put many of them off the whole business. The average modern girl and young mum doesn't want to push and poke her breasts and nipples about for months on end before the baby's even born!

There is *no* convincing evidence from all the surveys done so far that any ante-natal care – such as wearing breast shells (shields), rolling the nipples, doing nipple exercises, rubbing the nipples with a rough towel, putting on lanolin, cream or alcohol, expressing colostrum, etc – *does any good at all*! Having said this, though, we have to admit that there are some women who may be so squeamish that were it not for this breast preparation they might not feed their babies because of their reluctance to handle their own breasts. In these cases breast care might 'decondition' them sufficiently for them to manage breastfeeding.

There are three things that *are* worth talking about:

1 Nipple shape

Some women have nipples that don't stick out normally but seem to be flat or even inverted. If the areola of a nipple like this is pressed between the finger and thumb, and the nipple then sticks out properly, it's unlikely that the baby will later have any difficulty in sucking. Similarly, if your nipples stick out when you are sexually excited, you'll be all right when breastfeeding. However, if the nipples remain flat or inverted, there may be a problem later. To get things into perspective, though, 'poor' nipple shape hinders only one mother in twenty trying to feed her first baby; one in fifty feeding her second baby; and no mothers who have fed two babies or more.

When the finger-thumb areola test is done ante-natally, it suggests that one woman in three pregnant for the first time has 'poor' nipples (either truly inverted or just poorly protractile). So why the discrepancy with the numbers given above? It's because nipple shape and protractility improve spontaneously during pregnancy and this is thought to be because of the action of oestrogens on the tissues behind the nipple.

It's possible you'll be told you should wear breast shells (shields) if your nipples are too flat. These are hollow, plastic or glass, and saucer-shaped with a circular hole on the inner surface for the nipple, and of course they come in pairs. The idea behind them is that by wearing them inside your bra, your nipples will be pressed through the holes and this will improve their shape. They don't show when in position and are usually quite comfortable.

It's doubtful, though, whether wearing breast shells will definitely improve the protractility of the nipples. The nipples that do improve with shells probably would have done so naturally during pregnancy anyway, as we've just described. However, if you have poorly protractile nipples and you're determined to do everything possible to make sure you can feed easily, then wearing breast shells ante-natally inside your bra certainly won't hurt. When ordering or buying, ask for a pair of *breast shields*. We have called them breast shells in the book to differentiate them more clearly from nipple shields, and indeed they are widely known as shells, but they are manufactured under the name of breast shields.

Perhaps a better use for breast shells is after the baby is born, when their use for a time before a feed will often make the nipple protrude enough for the baby to be able to take hold of the breast properly. Obviously, after a few seconds or so the nipple returns to its original shape, so the baby has to catch hold fairly quickly. The disadvantage of this method is that the shell can obstruct milk ducts because of the pressure it exerts and so can increase the likelihood of engorgement. Also, the nipple skin can become moist and swollen in the shell and so more liable to become sore and cracked.

Many ante-natal clinics routinely look at nipples and advise mothers if they are poorly shaped. However, if they are it's no good just looking, so if someone only does this you can be sure that their advice won't be worth listening to. If after doing the finger-thumb test they advise you to wear breast shells, then do so if you want to but remember the benefit from doing so is unproven. If they say your nipples are fine, then at least you'll be reassured. If they don't examine your nipples at all, it shouldn't worry you. If you think your nipples are poorly shaped you can always ask next time and get them to order you breast shells if this would put your mind at rest. Remember that only 5 per cent of first-time mothers have any trouble with their nipples being 'unsuitable' for feeding which is scarcely surprising since this is what they were designed for.

2 Nipple cleanliness

The thing to understand here is that the Montgomery's tubercles around the areola secrete a greasy fluid which keeps the skin of the areola and nipple supple and also kills surface bacteria on the skin. If you wash this fluid off with soap, then the skin is much more likely to become sore when you suckle your baby. It doesn't matter how you wash your breasts for most of your pregnancy but keep away from soap for the last few weeks. Just wash your nipples by splashing them with warm water.

There's no need to use any sort of ointment or cream on your nipples to prepare them for breastfeeding – nature's own lubrication is best. Similarly, there's no need to remove any dried secretions from the nipple. A simple water splash is enough.

3 Expression of milk

There's no need to express milk ante-natally to remove colostrum or 'clear the ducts' as was once advised. However, it's worth learning the technique even though you won't actually use it now, because it may be useful to know when you've got the baby (see Chapter 7 for details).

What about all the other things that people tell you to do? It has been shown that 'rolling' the nipples doesn't increase success with feeding. The only reason for doing it would be to make your nipples less sensitive and that will happen anyway once the baby starts feeding. Some women go without their bra or cut a small hole in their bra each side to allow their nipples to rub against their clothing and so become less sensitive. Others rub their nipples with a rough towel each night after their bath, which seems rather hard on them! It also can't be shown to do any good.

So all you need to do ante-natally is clean your nipples with water alone; learn how to express milk to save you learning later; and, if you want to, use breast shells if your nipples are poorly protractile.

Eating the right food

The weight you'll gain during pregnancy is composed of the baby, the placenta, the amniotic fluid and the increased weight of the uterus and breasts, together with the increased amount of blood and other body fluids and stores of fat. Controversy rages over the amount of weight gain desirable.

A normal woman eating an unrestricted diet will gain on average twenty-eight pounds during pregnancy, of which about nine pounds will be made up of fat stores. If she bottle-feeds her baby, she may have trouble losing all this excess fat but if she breastfeeds, the fat contributes nourishment to the baby via the milk and is used up over the breastfeeding period provided she doesn't overeat. Recent research suggests that the fat stores accumulated during pregnancy supply about 300 calories a day to the baby in milk for about three or four months. Given that a baby needs to get around 600 to 800 calories a day from milk, this means that the breastfeeding mother has to eat only 300 to 500 extra calories a day (provided she has laid down adequate fat stores) in order to provide food for her baby without robbing her own body. This means that the fat she has stored during pregnancy provides between a third and a half of the baby's energy needs. Millions of women in developing countries don't lay down any fat stores yet still manage to breastfeed successfully for long periods, provided they have enough to eat.

Many obstetricians advise a weight gain of less than the average twenty-eight pounds and while this may be fine for the bottle-feeding mother, the breastfeeding mother will have to compensate for her lack of fat stores by eating more while she's breastfeeding. Too high a weight gain during pregnancy can make a woman's life unpleasant because she's more likely to have trouble with ankle swelling, varicose veins, backache and heartburn, so don't think that the more weight you put on, the better!

Studies to try to correlate success in breastfeeding with the weight gained during pregnancy have yielded conflicting results, one showing that the smaller the amount of fat stored, the greater the amount of milk produced, and another showing that women putting on very little weight during pregnancy had difficulty in feeding their babies. Clearly, more work needs to be done in this field.

So what should you eat? Eat a normal, balanced, healthy diet such as you should eat even when you're not pregnant. There's absolutely no need to eat for two! At the beginning of your pregnancy you may find you want to eat less than usual because of sickness but later you'll probably find that your appetite increases. Overall, you'll need slightly more food than usual to supply the needs of the growing baby and experts suggest a figure of an extra 200 calories a day. However, if like many women you're less active during the last few months of pregnancy, you may not need to eat any more at all.

A normal diet should contain enough protein, fluid, fat, and unrefined carbohydrate, including wholemeal flour products such as wholemeal bread, wholewheat cereals, brown rice, and fruit and vegetables. Fruit and vegetables should be unpeeled if possible and cooked as little as necessary. Added sugar in any form is best avoided as not only is it quite unnecessary for a healthy diet but it is also very high in calories and bad for your teeth. By eating unrefined food you will probably avoid any trouble with constipation – a common problem in pregnancy.

Provided you eat a well-balanced diet, there's no need for you to take any vitamin supplements.

Many people believe that milk is essential for the pregnant woman but this is quite untrue, provided she has enough calcium from other foods and that her diet is adequate overall. Calcium-containing foods include bread, cabbage, liver, watercress, fish and cheese. It's important to take at least some of these foods as the baby needs quite a lot of calcium for bone development and may otherwise rob your own bones of this vital substance. It's important to get this in perspective, though, by looking at many parts of the world where women do not increase their calcium intake during pregnancy and yet have healthy babies and remain healthy themselves.

Many doctors routinely give iron and folic acid supplements to pregnant women. This is to try to prevent the anaemia from deficiency of either of these substances which occurs in a small percentage of pregnant women. The World Health Organisation has recommended that there is no need for women in developed countries to take these supplements provided they are eating a balanced diet. Indeed, many women don't take them anyway as the side-effects of iron can be so unpleasant. Routine blood tests should be done during pregnancy (usually at the first visit and again at thirty-two weeks) to make sure that should true anaemia develop, it can be treated before the baby is born. Old estimates of the numbers of women developing anaemia didn't take into account the fact that the normal woman's haemoglobin concentration in her blood falls during pregnancy as a result of the increased amount of fluid in the blood – this of course is not the same as iron deficiency anaemia. To guard against anaemia you should eat enough foods containing iron (meat, eggs, green vegetables and wholemeal bread) and folic acid (green vegetables, liver, kidneys and yeast).

We'll talk about the ideal diet for a breastfeeding mother in Chapter 9 but it differs very little from the one we've just described.

So by now you should have everything prepared for breastfeeding and be looking forward to the birth of your baby. The next chapter will tell you exactly how to manage from the very first few minutes after birth.

7 The early days

Childbirth

A good obstetrician or midwife is a safe one. He or she is also one who stands back while the vast majority of women labour spontaneously and naturally, with no intervention. However, at the slightest suspicion of trouble he or she quietly and quickly steps forward to intervene in the labour so as to end up with a live, healthy mother and baby. Today, there is mounting research evidence that the average normal labour is easier for the mother and safer for the baby if the mother labours for most of the time in the first and second stages in an upright position. Also, she is much less likely to need an episiotomy (a surgical cut of her vaginal opening). Why is this important for breastfeeding? Because the better a mother feels after her labour, the easier it is for the breastfeeding relationship to get off to a good start. Also, if her contractions are easy to handle, she's less likely to ask for pain-killers, which can themselves cause problems for the breastfeeding baby after birth.

The first few minutes

The moment of birth comes not only at the end of many hours of hard labour but also at the end of nine months' waiting and preparation for the baby's arrival. Not surprisingly, the majority of mothers experience a tremendous sense of physical relief and emotional excitement when the baby is finally born. Feelings of pride at having actually produced a baby that a few hours ago was nothing more than a wriggling bump mingle with fatigue, curiosity and a sense of elation. A few mothers are so exhausted by their labour that all they can think of is having a well-earned rest and unfortunately some are so knocked out by the effects of pain-killing drugs that they can't think of anything at all.

Excessive doses of pain-killers during labour (especially drugs such as pethidine) are probably responsible for more breastfeeding failure than people have realised. It has been shown that animals anaesthetised while they give birth often reject their young and many mothers say they feel that the baby isn't quite real after giving birth under anaesthetic or under the influence of large amounts of pain-killing drugs. A mother's attachment to her baby will undoubtedly be delayed if she is overdosed with pain-killing drugs and she will be less likely to breastfeed successfully.

Research has shown that those babies born to 'over-doped' mothers don't develop normal feeding patterns until the fourth or fifth day! It's hardly surprising that with a difficult feeder on her hands a mother may become dispirited and give up. See page 170 for some ideas on how to cope.

Here then is a perfect opportunity for your husband to help. He can ensure that you don't get given too much in the way of pain-killers. Accept an injection only if you feel you really need it. Gas and air are probably a safer way of getting pain relief (from the baby's point of view) than injections of pethidine or similar powerful drugs.

Ideally, a new baby should be handed to his mother straight away to hold and suckle for as long as she wants. If the baby is naked, so much the better, as long as the room is warm enough. Staff permitting, weighing and washing can be done later.

In many obstetric units the newborn baby is wrapped up and handed to the mother to hold for a time before being weighed, washed and labelled. At the same time, the placenta is delivered and preparations for any stitches are made. It takes a single-minded mother to put her baby to the breast amid all this activity but we strongly recommend that she does because it'll give both her and her baby the best possible start to breastfeeding. Some mothers are so delighted with their new babies that immediate suckling seems perfectly normal and not at all embarrassing, even though there is a lot of activity around and it may be the first time they have suckled a baby. Other mothers are not really sure what's expected of them and feel awkward if the baby seems uninterested in the breast.

It has been suggested that the oxytocin secreted by the pituitary gland into the bloodstream during the first episode of suckling helps expel the placenta and reduce blood loss by its action on the uterus (it makes the muscle fibres contract). Indeed, some people use suckling as their only means of encouraging delivery of the afterbirth. Early suckling is certainly well worth doing because the sucking reflex of the newborn baby is strongest in the first half hour after birth, after which the baby often becomes tired and uninterested in the breast for a time.

Suckling before the umbilical cord is cut has the effect of pushing more blood along the cord into the baby as the uterus contracts. This 'extra helping' of iron-containing blood builds up the iron stores of the baby and so has much to recommend it. Early suckling means that many women won't need a routine injection of ergometrine to make their uterus contract and so detach the placenta and push it out. The cord can be cut as soon as the placenta has detached itself inside the uterus. (Your midwife or doctor can tell when this has happened.)

Waiting a few minutes until this happens instead of cutting the cord as soon as the baby is born means that the baby's life-line to his mother's blood supply is there a little longer and the need to get him breathing is not so urgent. As soon as the baby is breathing, he is getting his own oxygen supply, of course, and the cord can be cut straight away. If the placenta is detached and the baby still isn't breathing, the cord should be cut quickly and the baby given normal medical assistance. Without ergometrine, the placenta may take up to half an hour to be expelled naturally and during this time the mother can be getting to know her baby. All drugs are best avoided by the breastfeeding mother, and although it has not been proven, there is a suspicion that in certain circumstances ergometrine might reduce the milk supply.

It has been shown in four separate worldwide studies that early contact with her newborn baby makes a mother more likely to breastfeed successfully and also increases the length of time she'll continue to feed. It seems that there is a 'sensitive period' probably lasting about twelve hours which is important (though not essential) for the development of mother–child bonding. If the mother and child are separated for this period then the mother's behaviour towards the child may differ not only with respect to breastfeeding but also in the amount of affection she shows on the second day. All this means that the priority shouldn't be to take the baby away and give the mother time to sleep but should be to let mother and baby be together. A mother's sleep is more likely to be deep if she has looked at, cuddled and suckled her baby than if she is worrying about where he is and what is happening to him. Lots of mothers anyway aren't sleepy, especially after an undrugged delivery, but just want to talk about what has happened and have the baby there. It's difficult to take a pride in a baby who is taken away!

Have a good look at your baby and enjoy your first meeting. You may well not feel any rush of motherly love – some mothers say that this takes time to come, but at least you'll be curious to examine and touch him. Stroke or cuddle your baby if you want to. He'll have a distinctive smell and many newly delivered mothers comment on how delightful this smell is. Uncover your breast one side and see if your baby wants to feed. If he does, then let him carry on as long as he wants. It's all too easy to be discouraged by a baby that doesn't seem very interested but remember that he doesn't yet know what he should suck. When he has tasted your colostrum he'll be much keener!

What's the best way to put the newborn baby to the breast? If you're lying down, roll to one side and lay the baby down by you so that he's on his side with his head facing your breast. Then stroke his cheek or the corner of his mouth with your nipple. He may open his mouth as he turns towards your nipple and then start feeding when he finds it. This searching movement is called *rooting* and is an inborn reflex in newborn babies. Don't hold his head or push it towards the breast or he'll turn his mouth towards the pressure of your hand and that will be the opposite way from the way you want him to turn! Many babies like to gaze at their mothers and are in no hurry for the breast. They may get excited and lick the nipple or just hold it in their mouths and the sucking comes later. It's interesting that the focal length of a new baby's eyes is approximately the same as the distance between his eyes and his mother's when he is at her breast.

If you can sit up comfortably, then hold the baby in the crook of one arm, make sure you're comfortable, preferably with your elbow supported, and do what we've just described. If the baby is comfortable, with his whole body facing yours, not just with his head turned to your breast, then he's more likely to feed (see also page 91).

Don't worry if you feel inexperienced or at a loss how to hold and behave with your baby. This is quite normal, especially if it's your first time. You won't know instantly how to do it right. Studies with animals show that they too need time and experience to become good at mothering. Some zoo animals need to be taught how to 'mother' by male keepers!

So far we've been talking about the average mother who has had a normal labour. This doesn't always happen, though, and we'll talk about the mother who has had a Caesarean section or other problems in Chapter 13.

So what happens next? Ideally, if you, your husband and your baby are all content, the staff will leave you together for a while – perhaps half an hour or so. After that you'll be washed and given clean things to wear and the baby can have all the necessary routine things done.

Rooming-in

Enlightened hospitals allow the baby to sleep in your bed or in a cot by you and to be with you all the time, knowing that you'll sleep better and be happier with your baby by you day and night. Studies show that mothers who have their babies with them are twice as likely to succeed at breastfeeding than if their babies are in a nursery. After all, you've had him with you for nine months and there's no good reason to take him away now. Although it is still a rare occurrence, some hospitals 'allow' mothers to have their babies in bed with them all the time. This works very well for mothers, babies and the nursing staff, even in a large ward.

In general it's fair to say that no hospital can possibly have enough staff to give a baby the kind of love and care that his mother can give. It's scarcely surprising then that babies who room in are more contented than those kept in nurseries and brought to their mothers occasionally.

Even mothers cared for in large, open post-natal wards can have their babies by them at night, provided they pick them up as soon as they need a cuddle or a feed to avoid waking other mothers. Rooming-in makes life much easier for the staff, pleasanter for both mothers and babies, and leads to far less noise because the babies don't have to cry. Mothers sleep better knowing that they don't have to worry about whether their baby is crying untended in the nursery or is being given a bottle.

If you feel very strongly about having your baby with you at night but the hospital staff are not keen, ask your husband to join with you in insisting on it.

Breast milk only

If your baby is taken away from you, ensure that he is brought to you for feeding as soon as he cries and that he is *not given anything to drink*, even if it's only water or sugar water. Don't be fobbed off with explanations or excuses – he's your baby and, as we've already explained earlier in this chapter, the best way to establish successful lactation is to feed him frequently in the first few days. If he has anything else to drink, he won't want to feed at the breast.

Many mothers have described the agony they went through when they could hear their babies crying and yet weren't allowed to have them brought to them. What some nurses don't understand is that a mother doesn't know the sound of her baby's voice this soon after birth and so worries every time *any* baby cries. She'll have far more peace of mind with her baby by her. Her milk will also come in far sooner if she picks up the baby to feed him not only whenever he cries but also whenever she wants to.

Hospital staff may ask why it is that *your* baby is not allowed to drink cows' milk formula, sugar water or boiled water at night (or when you are asleep) when every other baby has it and seems to get on well enough. Tell them that there are many reasons why breast milk alone is best. If it makes things easier, here's a list.

1 The more your baby feeds, the sooner your milk will come in.

2 Your breasts need to be emptied frequently to produce plenty of milk. Infrequent feeding will diminish your milk supply.

3 Your baby needs colostrum to protect him from infection, to give him the foods he needs in the correct proportions, to supply him with immunoglobulins and other substances not present in cows' milk formula and to encourage his bowel to expel its sticky contents (meconium).

4 Your baby shouldn't have cows' formula milk because this would satiate his appetite for several hours and so make him less likely to want breast milk. The bottle-fed baby goes longer

between feeds than the breastfed baby because cows' milk takes longer to be digested.

5 Your baby shouldn't have cows' milk formula because it contains 'foreign' protein which might sensitise him if he's susceptible and so predispose him to allergy later.

6 He needn't have sugar water because your own milk will provide all the sugar and water a healthy baby needs. A high calorie drink would anyway satiate his appetite and once again prevent him from wanting to feed at the breast. A sudden slug of sugar is completely unphysiological and unnatural, so why give it?

7 Properly breastfed babies don't need water. Your breast milk has enough even in the first days. Research done at the University of Rochester (New York) showed that if breastfed babies were given water or cows' milk formula complements in the first few days of life, they lost more weight and were less likely to start gaining before they left hospital than if they were entirely breastfed. (The same, incidentally, went for bottle-fed babies given water.)

8 He shouldn't be fed with a bottle and a teat. A rubber teat is so easy for the baby to drink from and provides such a strong stimulus to suck that the baby may be loath to return to your breast when he finds he has to work harder to get his milk from you.

Hospitals sometimes used to recommend that all babies had water or sugar water as their first drink in case there was a congenital abnormality of their windpipe and gullet and milk was inhaled. This is now no longer justified.

Sleeping and night feeds

During your hospital stay it's ideal if your baby can be in your bed or in a cot by you at night but if he has to go into a nursery then make sure that you tell the nurses each night that you are breastfeeding. Although they should know, it's easy to get a young nurse who is inexperienced, an agency nurse who is new, or a nurse who thinks she is doing you a favour, who will not bring your baby to you to be fed but will give him a bottle of cows' milk formula, sugar water or water along with all the other bottle-fed babies at two a.m. Some mothers who have been warned about this write out a card which they tie on to their baby's cot. The card says, 'I am breastfed – please take me to my mother when I cry.' This won't upset anybody and will probably make it easier for you to get your own way, though it's not infallible. It's worth getting yourself mentally geared up to night feeds because you'll be doing plenty of them. Night feeds may decrease from two months or so but many babies are loath to give them up for many months or even years.

Young babies have more periods of light, REM (rapid eye movement) sleep than do older children and adults, and it is during these periods that they are most likely to wake for a feed. As he gets older, your baby will have longer periods of deeper sleep and will be less likely to wake up.

Try to get as much sleep as you can between feeds during the first days especially as labour is a tiring experience for most mothers and broken nights also take their toll.

The nursing staff may suggest that you rest lying on your tummy for an hour or so every day. This position is uncomfortable if your breasts are at all full but you can make yourself quite comfy if you lie with your head on one pillow with another pillow below your breasts so as to make a sort of bridge.

You may be too excited to sleep much after your baby is born. It's a common feeling to want to live right through the whole birth experience over and over again in your mind, as though you were learning it. Some mothers find that they dream very little in the first few days or weeks after the birth, probably because their sleep patterns are being broken by the baby waking for feeds. Sleeping with the baby by your side means that you soon get used to snoozing through his feeding times, even though you may not be properly asleep.

How often should you feed?

Feed your baby whenever he cries; when he seems to want feeding; when your breasts are full; and more often if you want to. *Don't feed on any sort of schedule.* The more schedule feeding there has been this century, the fewer breastfeeding mothers there have been. Schedules reduce the likelihood of successful breastfeeding. We've already shown why this is so in Chapter 2. However, while demand feeding works perfectly well for many mothers and their babies, it's not necessarily the best way of feeding a baby because he may not ask for enough feeds. In this case your milk supply will dwindle. *Natural breastfeeding doesn't necessarily mean waiting until your baby asks. You may want to feed him at other times because your breasts are full, just before going out, because you simply want to cuddle him or because he is jaundiced, tired, affected by your drugs in labour, ill, pre-term, small for dates, or apathetic and not asking for enough feeds.* In any case, don't leave your baby unfed for more than three hours at the longest – longer gaps will endanger your milk supply and may mean your baby is not getting enough food. Some mothers find their babies go as long as four or five hours between some feeds but as a general rule this is not sensible in the early days.

Demand feeding is usually held to be the ideal form of breast-feeding – which it certainly is when compared with schedule feeding. But it's still not as good as natural breastfeeding where both mother's and baby's needs are met whenever they want.

Babies gain weight better when fed frequently because their mothers produce more milk. Many people have worked out the average number of feeds demanded by babies each day after birth and this number varies a lot, according to the individual baby. Don't worry about the number of feeds your baby has compared with the demand-fed baby in the next bed – it doesn't matter and is no indication of the success you'll have. All babies are different.

So for that matter are mothers. Don't compare yourself with the other women around you even if they're breastfeeding. Obviously it's interesting to know how many feeds your neighbour's baby has but the danger is that you'll start competing with each other. This is one reason why mothers breastfeed more successfully if they go home soon after delivery.

You may find that the nurses on your ward will be unwilling to let you feed on demand because it doesn't fit into their routine. It'll help if you tell them that research in a hospital in Oxford found that the nurses' work fell dramatically when the ward changed from schedule to demand breastfeeding.

Babies allowed absolutely unrestricted access to their mother's breasts – for example those carried next to a naked breast all day in some developing countries – don't have to cry before they are fed. These babies feed *very much more often* than babies fed even completely on demand in the western world. This is true natural breastfeeding.

Anthropologists tell us that it's possible to predict how often the young of any mammal will want to be suckled by the amount of protein in the milk. If the milk contains a lot of protein (as does that of the cow or some species of rabbit), then the young want to be suckled only infrequently – perhaps once a day. However, if the milk is low in protein, then the young need to be suckled very often. Human milk has very low levels of protein and we are grouped along with other mammals with low protein milk *as 'continuous contact mammals'*. Human babies will suck on and off for much of the time, given the chance, and this seems to be what Nature intended. The frequency of feeding can be reduced simply by not carrying our babies next to our naked breasts all day and by not sleeping naked next to them at night! However, if we make feeds too infrequent, we run the dual risk of reducing the milk supply through too little breast stimulation, and of separating our babies from ourselves too much, so not giving them enough physical and emotional comfort.

Some mothers worry about waking their babies during the daytime in order to feed them. You ought to wake your baby if it's a long time since a feed or if your breasts are feeling full. If you don't you'll regret it (and so will he in the end) because your breasts will become tense or even engorged and your milk production will slow down. Your baby will soon go back to sleep again so don't worry about waking him. After all, you're a nursing pair – sometimes you'll feed for his benefit and sometimes for yours. As the weeks go by your supply will tune in to his needs but in the meantime a few extra feeds will do no harm. As a general rule, you should never go so long between feeds that your breasts feel tense and lumpy.

Finally, mothers of naturally breastfed babies are only half as likely to get sore nipples and engorgement as those of schedule-fed babies (see also pages 94 and 157).

How long should feeds be?

You'll almost certainly be told to feed your baby for a specified number of minutes each side and to increase the time each day until the fifth day when you'll be 'allowed' ten minutes a side. *This restriction of feeding time is not only completely unnatural but will hinder your milk from coming in; may not give your let-down reflex time to work and become established; will prevent your baby from getting as much colostrum as he could get; and will make you much more likely to get sore nipples*. This has all been known for years but some hospitals still insist on out-of-date rules.

Babies, like adults, want different amounts of food from day to day and even within any given day. Sometimes your baby will want a snack and other times a feast. Research done recently in southern Africa has shown that any given baby feeding on demand will take meals of very different volumes at different times. Sometimes one feed is ten times as big as another.

If you're not the sort of person to question the rules openly, and few women are when they've just had a baby, then go ahead and suckle for as long as you want anyway.

Let your baby feed till he's had enough. Once he loses interest in the first breast, change him to the second. Always try to feed from both breasts in the early days or the unemptied one will produce less milk because of back-pressure on the milk-producing cells.

Start the next feed with the breast you fed with last because the let-down is more efficient early in a breastfeed. The first breast is therefore usually emptied better than the second and it's important for both breasts to take turns at being emptied (see also page 110).

How to tell when he's had enough

Many babies show they've had enough simply by falling asleep but before that stage a baby may well unclench his fists, smile, show obvious refusal or arch his back. Don't force him to feed more. Learn to accept your baby's judgement of what he wants. After a while you'll get to know how much he's had by feeling your breasts. Lots of babies like to doze on and off during a feed, especially if they are pre-term.

What about stopping him feeding?

Some babies simply let the nipple go when they've had enough to drink whilst others have to be gently removed from the breast or they'll be there all day, sucking in their sleep. If your nipples are sore you may have to limit your baby's time at the breast for a day or two. Be sure not to do this for too long or your milk supply will fall off.

Never pull your baby's mouth away from the breast while he's feeding. This can damage the nipple and areola as the strong negative pressure is broken. It is better to break the pressure by putting the tip of your little finger in the corner of his mouth. He will then come easily and painlessly away from the nipple.

Crying

There's an awful lot going on in the average maternity ward, what with trolley shops, paper rounds, meals, visitors, bed-making and room cleaning, to say nothing of doctors' and nurses' rounds, flowers to arrange, letters and cards to open and send, baths, talking to your neighbour in the next bed and so on. It's all too easy to let the baby come second while you go on doing whatever you were doing when he started crying. Remember that if you leave him crying for long, he'll get tired out because infants expend a lot of energy crying – just look and you'll see why. When your baby has been crying for a long time you'll probably find he doesn't feed well – he has literally exhausted himself with crying and hasn't got the strength to feed.

At first you won't have a clue why he's crying and this can make any new mother feel inadequate but it's the only way he can communicate. After a few weeks you may be able to distinguish his cries between hunger, tiredness, a dirty bottom and so on.

Long periods of crying are one of the main reasons why babies fed on a four-hourly schedule don't get enough breast milk and why their mothers often fail with breastfeeding. A baby who wakes an hour early and is left to cry until the clock says it is time for a feed won't be hungry when feed time arrives – he'll just be tired out. Over a few days his mother's breasts won't have been stimulated enough because she won't have suckled enough so there won't be enough prolactin and oxytocin released (see Chapter 2) and her milk supply will fail.

There are two other reasons why babies shouldn't be left to cry. Firstly, no mother likes to hear her baby crying – crying means unhappiness to most people. This will upset her even if she pretends it doesn't and her let-down reflex (see Chapter 2) may easily be suppressed as a result.

Secondly, it seems sensible to comfort a squawling infant straight away as this will encourage him to think that mother is good and that the world is a good place to be in. You can't possibly spoil a baby like this. If you were left to yell for hours for your food you would be angry; babies are no different.

Many mothers have commented on how babies brought up to be

comforted (and fed) at the breast whenever they cry grow up to be happy, independent, loving children – not demanding, unhappy, spoilt ones.

The ability to comfort her crying baby at the breast is one of the greatest pleasure for the breastfeeding mother. If she limits suckling time this pleasure will be denied to both her and her baby. Breastfeeding is not only a means of getting milk: it's also a way of being close to a warm, soft, comforting mother (see also page 109).

How to hold your baby

If you can, experiment with various positions by yourself. If you've got someone who is in a hurry or unsympathetic standing by you, pushing and prodding the baby, neither you nor your baby will be relaxed and the feed is unlikely to go well. We've talked briefly about feeding the baby sitting up or lying down after delivery (see page 82). The main things are to make yourself comfortable (because you'll be feeding for some time) and to get the baby comfortable. Don't hold the back of his head but let his head rest on your arm. Try supporting his weight with a pillow on your lap. If your supporting arm is taking his weight, sooner or later you'll end up with aching shoulders and back. If you're relaxed physically, it's easier to relax mentally, which means that your milk will let down more readily. Position yourself and the baby so that it's as easy as possible for him to take the nipple and some of the areola into his mouth. If you're sitting it's easier if you are sitting upright and perhaps leaning forward slightly. Try holding the baby with his chest and tummy against you so that he doesn't have to turn his head round but can feed with his head straight. Some babies like it best if they have something to hold on to – try giving him your finger. Many mothers find that as soon as their baby has had enough he lets go of whatever he's holding.

Don't push his mouth on to your nipple as the rooting reflex will make him turn towards your hand. Just stroke the side of his mouth with your nipple and offer him the nipple and with luck he'll latch on. Some babies have such a strong rooting reflex that they turn their heads to feed even if a sheet or some clothing touches their cheek. Others need help to get them latched on. If your breast is very full you may have to hold it back so that his nose isn't smothered, otherwise you don't have to hold your nipple or breast once he's feeding unless it's easier. Expressing a little milk from a full breast will soften it enough to enable the baby to latch on.

Your nipple and as much of the areola as possible should be taken into the baby's mouth as the milk reservoirs are under the areola and need to be emptied by the baby's mouth movements. If only the nipple goes in, not enough milk will be drawn out and because the baby is not getting enough milk he'll suck very strongly and may make your nipple sore. If you have a very large areola which the baby finds difficult to take into his mouth, try holding it between your finger and thumb or between your index and middle fingers (the cigarette hold) and squeezing them together. This will make the areola flatter (like a biscuit) and easier for him to take. A good principle is to aim the nipple up to the baby's nose once it's in his mouth – this will ensure it's in the best position (high up in the mouth) and will not get hurt when he sucks on it.

But most important of all is to relax as you feed. Think back to your relaxation teaching from ante-natal classes and relax every muscle you can. Enjoy your baby as he feeds and don't let anything put you off this happy, relaxed state of mind. If you're happier with curtains drawn round the bed, ask someone to draw them for you. If anyone makes adverse comments about the baby not feeding well, take their advice but tell them calmly that you've all the time in the world to learn. Remember that a baby can safely go the first few days without much to drink – nature intended him to have only small amounts of colostrum from you.

A difference you may notice between your baby and a bottle-fed one is that your baby doesn't feed continuously. He may stop feeding every so often and look around. This is because the let-down causes milk to be spurted into the ducts and from the nipple in an uneven flow. Several spurts of milk come out and then there is a short pause before milk is again ejected. Your baby is just adapting to the flow of your milk. His breathing pattern is adjusted to fit in with his drinking pattern.

Even a newborn baby may stare at you fixedly from time to time, or even all the time. It's a wonderful feeling having a baby gazing up at you from your breast, so enjoy it and also take time to admire and stroke him, provided you don't put him off his sucking for too long. It's all too easy to become so intent on doing everything 'properly' that you don't spend any time simply enjoying being close to your baby. Sometimes you could undress your baby (in a warm room) and hold him close to your naked body. You can feed him like this if you like, with nappies in strategic places to soak up leaks from you and him!

Don't forget that a baby can be at the breast quite comfortably while you are sitting, lying on one side, or standing, though it's not so comfortable standing because you have to support all his weight (unless you're clever with a babysling). You may like to cuddle and wash your baby in the bath with you when you are having a bath. Babies often much prefer this to being washed in a baby bath as they can be held securely in their mother's arms and can also be put to the breast if they want. Make sure the water is at a suitable temperature for the baby and bear in mind that bathing with your baby is easier if someone is there to hand him to you and take him from you.

Some mothers enjoy massaging their babies all over with warm oil and the babies enjoy it too.

The important thing to remember is that there are no limits to the amount of time you and your baby can spend together and that babies thrive on lots of body contact, love and attention.

Old but still widely practised customs are swaddling or wrapping babies securely in a piece of material such as a soft sheet or shawl. Towards the end of pregnancy babies are held fairly tightly by the walls of the uterus and swaddling perhaps reminds them of the security of being inside their mothers. Certainly babies carried next to their mothers all day are held firmly by the sling or length of material used and they seem to like it. If your baby has gone to sleep after a feed and you want to put him down, wrap him snugly and firmly in a soft sheet, with his arms and legs inside. He's less likely to wake with a startle if you do this and he'll be nice and warm too.

What is he getting?

At first your baby gets colostrum which provides him with many essential nutrients. This colostrum gradually changes into mature milk during the first few days. There is no sudden change. The more a baby feeds, the sooner milk will be produced in large amounts and when this happens it's known as the milk 'coming in'. In a mother feeding her baby frequently, the milk may come in on the second or third day after birth. In a mother feeding her baby infrequently, it may not come in until the fourth or fifth day.

Obviously the sooner the milk comes in, the sooner the baby will get plenty to drink. The mother having her second baby will find that her milk comes in sooner than it did with her first.

The phrase 'the milk coming in' is misleading in that it has led many people to think that before the milk comes in, the breasts are empty. Of course they aren't, as you can see if you express some colostrum. Colostrum is produced only in fairly small amounts. *It's meant to be this way* and even very small volumes are worth their weight in gold to the baby. So valuable is colostrum in protecting the newborn baby against infections (among other things) that some experts believe that every bottle-fed baby should receive a 'colostrum cocktail'. Farmers have been giving this to their valuable calves for years.

Never doubt your ability to nourish your baby in these first few days. Your colostrum may not look much but cows' milk formula, in however large a volume, cannot compare with it for goodness.

Engorgement (swollen, tender breasts)
When the milk comes in you should carry on feeding your baby frequently so that you avoid getting engorged breasts. Mothers feeding their babies on a schedule are twice as likely to suffer from engorgement as those feeding on demand. If you are feeding your baby the natural way you're highly unlikely to get engorged.

Mothers who notice a large increase in the size of their breasts when their milk comes in often think that their milk supply must be failing when their breasts become smaller. However, the supply isn't failing (provided they are feeding their babies on demand), it's just that the breasts tend to revert to a smaller size once the milk supply equals the demand.

Turn to page 94 for details of treatment if your breasts actually become engorged.

Expressing milk
You may need to express some milk by hand in the first few days while your baby's needs are catching up with your supply and certainly expression is a useful technique to know for later just in case you need it. If your breasts become tense it may be difficult for the baby to grasp the nipple and areola. Expressing your milk will soften the breast enough to allow him to latch on.

If your baby is premature and as a result too immature to breastfeed, milk will have to be given via a tube. You can establish your milk supply by expressing milk at short, regular intervals – preferably every two or three hours – and this can be given to your baby by tube.

To express milk, first wash your hands, then hold the areola between your thumb and first finger. Some people find it easier to use the left hand for both breasts and to use the right hand to collect the milk in a container. If you intend to store the milk in a fridge or freezer, the container should be sterilised. Move your hand firmly backwards towards your chest. Now move your hand away, pressing your finger and thumb together, so gently squeezing milk out of the milk reservoirs under the areola. Even when milk is expressed it's still necessary for your let-down reflex to work for the hindmilk to be obtained. The milk will then come in spurts with intervals between and you should go on expressing even during the intervals to stimulate the let-down. Many women also massage the whole breast gently to encourage the milk flow. Change sides several times to encourage more milk to come. Don't forget that when your milk is let down, it'll drip or even spray from *both* breasts. If you're collecting the milk to give your baby and not just expressing some to relieve overfull breasts, remember to catch the milk from the other breast as well and not just from the one you're expressing at the time. Many mothers who donate milk to breast milk banks at their local hospitals collect the drips from the breast their baby is not feeding from. Such drips can easily be collected in a breast shell (shield) worn inside the bra cup. Breasts shells can be sterilised. Don't forget to put the shell inside your bra with the tiny hole uppermost! Pour the collected drips into a sterile bottle or other container that you can cover.

When expressing your milk it's important to express it from all parts of the breast. You will need to move your thumb and finger to several different positions to do this, and to use your other hand if necessary.

Expressing milk often takes longer than actually feeding the baby but is easy once you have the knack. Don't worry if you can express only a small amount. Most successful breastfeeders can never express more than one or two ounces at one go.

If you are expressing milk *after* you've fed your baby, perhaps because you want to leave breast milk in the fridge for a babysitter to give to your baby, don't be put off by the small amounts of milk which disappear. The fractions of an ounce soon mount up if you collect after each feed for a couple of days in advance of needing it. Don't forget to collect the milk that drips or sprays from the other breast when you're expressing or feeding your baby, using a breast shell inside your bra cup.

Storing milk

Having expressed the milk into a sterilised plastic container, cover the container and keep it in the fridge. Plastic is better than glass, as certain immunological components of milk stick to glass and are lost. You can freeze milk but this harms the living cells so don't keep it in the freezer unless really necessary. Having said this, frozen breast milk is still better than cows' milk formula.

It's sensible to freeze small amounts of milk because, once thawed, breast milk should not be refrozen so any left over will be wasted. You can always thaw more if it's needed. Thaw the milk quickly by holding the container under running water, first cold, then gradually warmer until the milk is liquid. You can then continue warming it in a pan of water on the stove. Milk at body temperature (slightly cool to your skin) is most pleasant for the baby. Pre-term babies should never have their milk cold.

Nipple care

In the old days the advice on preparing for a feed was so complicated that many mothers were heard to say that preparing their breasts for feeding was more fiddly than preparing bottles – so they chose bottles. Nipple and breast care is in fact easy.

There's no need to wash your breasts and nipples before a feed. When you have a bath, wash your nipples with water *but not* soap.

If you are told to put salt in the water to help heal your perineum, splash your breasts with plenty of plain water to remove the salt before you dry them. Don't let your nipples soak in the water as this will make them more liable to soreness and cracking.

There's no need to put anything on your nipples. Although lanolin or special creams such as Massé cream won't hurt, they are unnecessary as Montgomery's tubercles provide natural secretions. Your baby will also like the taste of you best.

It is suggested by many experienced breastfeeding mothers, though not proven, that nipple soreness can be prevented to some extent if a little milk is expressed when the baby has finished feeding, and rubbed over the nipples. Certainly there's no need to wash your breasts after a feed, though you could rinse them with water if you really want to. The smell of your milk, though imperceptible to outsiders, will attract your baby when you next put him to the breast. If he's a reluctant feeder, this could make all the difference to his desire to suck.

The nipple skin can easily become soggy and liable to crack if it's left moist. Avoid this by changing your breast pads often or, best of all, by leaving your bra off altogether so that your nipples are open to the air. This is most easily done at night.

This advice may sound rather complicated – all you need to do in fact is occasionally wash your breasts, avoid getting soap on the nipples and keep the nipples dry between feeds. That's all!

Nipple soreness and pain
Quite a few mothers experience soreness of their nipples during the first week or perhaps later. This seems to affect fair-skinned women with pale areolae more than darker-skinned women with dark areolae. Unfortunately, the pain makes many mothers give up breastfeeding – often because they're given wrong advice on how to cope with it.

By looking after your nipples as we've described above and by feeding naturally you may be able to prevent the onset of soreness. If you can't, then turn to page 157 for details of what to do.

Visiting
This can be a vexed subject. You feel left out if you don't have visitors when everyone else does; you want to show off your new baby to your relatives and friends; you may feel shy about feeding in front of people but yet don't want your baby to go hungry if he cries at visiting times; and a whole hour may be too much for you with some visitors but not enough with others.

There are several ways to cope. Try to choose a hospital that allows fairly unrestricted visiting and then get your husband to vet all the people who want to come and see you. If you wouldn't feel happy about feeding in front of them, ask him to put them off, tactfully, of course. There'll be plenty of other opportunities to see them.

Doing this will mean that you won't have to worry if your baby wants a feed during visiting – you'll just go ahead and do it. When people come to see you at home you can always go to another room to feed if you're embarrassed (or if you think they will be), but you can't do that in hospital.

Nappy changing

Many hospitals advise changing the baby's nappy before a feed. This is all very well if the baby isn't crying for a feed but if he is, wait till the end of the feed, otherwise you may be so upset that you won't let down your milk and your baby may be so upset that he regurgitates much of his feed after swallowing a lot of air between sobs. Some babies don't feed well with a wet or dirty nappy and others are woken by being changed after a feed, which is why changing before a feed is suggested. But after a good feed most babies are so content and full that nothing, not even a nappy change, will wake them. If you have one of those babies who won't feed in a dirty nappy, you'll soon find out and will have to change his nappy first.

A change after a feed would seem to make more sense because babies often wet or mess their nappy during a feed. For the baby who falls asleep halfway through a feed a nappy change will often wake him enough to take the second breast.

Baby's bowels

A breastfed baby's motions gradually change during the first week from the dark green meconium of the first day or so to the bright yellow, liquid motions which may be seen as only a stain on the nappy. Contrast this with a bottle-fed baby who has bulky motions almost as soon as he has got rid of the meconium.

In the early days of breastfeeding it's usual for almost every nappy to have a yellow stain on it.

Wind

Why haven't we mentioned winding yet? Because many breastfed babies don't need winding – they simply bring up any wind quite spontaneously or pass it out the other end. If you think your baby is windy, cuddle him in a fairly upright position, for instance up against your shoulder after a feed to let the wind come up. If you know that he doesn't usually burp, you can lay him down to sleep immediately after a feed. Wind is a subject that seems to have become an obsession with some mothers. Many countries of the world, including some European ones, don't recognise wind as being a problem and so do nothing about it.

There are some babies who are quite obviously uncomfortable after a feed but drop off to sleep when they've brought up some wind. Such babies sometimes frown or even go momentarily cross-eyed with the wind. You may notice that the skin above their upper lip is slightly blue and they may cry or fidget. If being upright doesn't do the trick, try sitting the baby on your lap with one of your hands rubbing his back gently and the other hand holding his chest. If you then bend him slightly in the middle, a bubble of air often comes up, perhaps with a little regurgitated milk. If you feed your baby lying down at night, you'll probably occasionally need to sit him up in bed to get rid of some swallowed air if he doesn't settle easily.

Colic

In strict medical terms colic is the intermittent pain caused by the involuntary contraction of smooth muscles in the walls of a hollow organ in the body, such as the colon.

Many babies cry for long periods during the day and especially in the evenings during the first three months. This crying is traditionally put down to 'evening colic' or 'three month colic' as it is also known. It is generally assumed that the 'colic' is caused by excess gas in the baby's bowels causing pain as it is passed through. There is, however, no evidence to prove that this is so because these babies have no more gas in their bowels – as shown on X-rays – than other babies, and it is highly likely that these bouts of crying are not due to colic at all. Other explanations include the baby being upset because his mother is overwrought with the evening rush of things to do – babies quickly sense and respond to moods; the baby being hungry because he is schedule-fed and allowed only ten minutes each side every few hours, even if his mother hasn't as much milk as at other feeds because she is tired; the baby has swallowed too much air while trying to drink fast-flowing milk (see pages 147 and 174); the baby may just want attention and cuddling at the time of day when his mother can't easily give it; the baby is allergic or sensitive to traces of foods that the mother has eaten present in her breast milk, e.g. cows' milk, alcohol, chocolate and cabbage; and lastly, it has been suggested that if the mother generally has her biggest meal in the evening, she may not be making milk of sufficient quantity or quality to satisfy the baby in the hours leading up to this meal.

The best way to cope with 'colic' is to relax and reduce the amount of work you are doing; feed the baby as much as he wants; just sit and cuddle him if he is happier like that (or get your husband to do the cuddling – some colicky babies quieten better with someone other than their mother); check what you have been eating; and make sure you eat regularly yourself. Drug treatment should then be unnecessary.

Some mothers believe that vitamin drops can give their babies colic. A trial of avoidance is easy to do if you suspect this. Another easy thing to try is holding your baby in different positions after a feed, for instance with him leaning slightly forwards and bending to the right, with your arm pressing against his abdomen. He'll assume this position if you hold him with his back to you, your arm round his right side and your right hand supporting his crotch.

Regurgitation (posseting)

Many babies, and small ones in particular, regurgitate milk during and after a feed, especially if the milk flow from the breast is very fast so that they swallow air as they attempt to swallow the milk, or if they are overfilled. Sometimes a baby will bring up so much milk that he will want more to drink to replace it.

There is no need to worry if your baby is thriving yet regurgitates milk like this. If your milk flow is very fast at first, though, you might try expressing some milk before feeding your baby, to prevent him having to drink it too quickly.

If the milk has been in your baby's tummy for some time, you'll notice that it has changed into fine curds and whey when it is brought up.

Afterpains

When your let-down reflex works, you may notice low tummy pains which are caused by oxytocin making your womb contract. It means not only that your womb is being encouraged to return to its former size but also that your let-down is working, which is heartening to know. Other signs that your let-down is working are tingling in the breasts, dripping or spraying of milk, the relief of nipple pain as the milk gets to the baby and the swallowing noises the baby makes (see also page 13).

Talking of pains, don't hesitate to tell the doctors or nurses if you're getting pain from episiotomy stitches, because there's nothing like a nagging pain from any source to put the dampers on the let-down reflex. Try something simple first like a hot bath and then ask for a rubber ring to sit on to take the weight off the most tender parts. If these simple measures don't work, ask for some pain-killers.

Leaking (see also page 14)

This will obviously happen if your let-down works before the baby is put to the breast but happens even without the let-down if your breasts are full, especially if you are warm and if you lean forward. Leaking means that your breasts are full and ready for the baby and ideally you should suckle your baby so as to relieve them, even if he doesn't seem hungry. If your breasts are full for too long, they're highly likely to become engorged in the first few weeks.

If you leak, don't worry that you're producing too much milk, because you're probably not. Don't cut down on your fluid intake in an effort to stop the leaking as this won't help. You can cope with leaking by using breast pads, soft material such as a handkerchief, an old terry nappy cut into squares, or a folded 'one-way' nappy liner tucked into your bra. A trick many mothers have discovered is to put the heel of one hand over the nipple and push it firmly towards the breast. This often stops the leaking like magic. To avoid soaking your nipple in soggy material while feeding from the first breast, try uncovering the second breast and letting the leaking milk drip on to a terry nappy. Soggy nipple skin, especially in the first few weeks, can make soreness and cracking much more likely.

Baby blues

Many newly delivered mothers feel weepy and emotional around the fourth day. This often coincides with the milk coming in and may be the result of the surging changes in hormones. It happens just as often in bottle-feeding mothers: in fact, probably more so. Unfortunately, if a mother is having any trouble in feeding her baby, this temporary depression may be the last straw that makes her decide to change to the bottle.

Apart from hormonal changes, it's not surprising that a newly delivered mother is emotional. Giving birth is a crisis point in a woman's life and the accompanying loss of sleep and the excitement surrounding a new baby are bound to upset even the calmest person to some extent. It's not uncommon for one mother in a ward to start crying and for all the others to follow suit. All the more reason, then, to learn how to cope with breastfeeding problems before you have your baby, so at least you haven't got that to worry about.

Modern hospital procedures that institutionalise and regiment women do little to help the fragile emotions of the new mother and depression can undoubtedly be made all the worse for those mothers whose babies are taken away from them and kept in nurseries. Simple kindness, praise, encouragement and sympathy on the part of the post-natal ward staff matter a great deal when you've just had a baby. Similarly, the slightest criticism can cause floods of tears.

Normal weight loss

A newborn baby has a lot of fluid in his body to tide him over the first few days when his mother's colostrum doesn't provide much volume.

The weight loss that is a perfectly normal occurrence in the first few days occurs because of the natural loss of fluid. Most babies lose 6 per cent of their body weight and many lose 10 per cent.

Weight gain

The speed at which a breastfed baby regains his birth weight depends to some extent on whether he is fed on a restricted basis or not. Babies fed on demand don't lose much weight after birth and have a more rapid weight gain than babies on a three-hourly feeding schedule. Babies on a three-hourly schedule do better than those on a four-hourly one.

In one study, 49 per cent of demand-fed babies and 36 per cent of four-hourly fed babies had regained their birth weight by a week. The demand-fed babies in this particular survey were, however, restricted in their number of feeds for the first two days; had they not been, there might have been even more babies regaining their birth weight at one week in this group. Some babies take up to three weeks to regain their birth weight and a few quite healthy ones take even longer.

But the speed at which birth weight is regained is not very important. In the old days a mother was not allowed to take her baby home until it had regained its birth weight and this still sometimes happens today. However, provided that the baby is being fed on an unrestricted basis; seems happy; his weight is slowly rising; the mother's let-down reflex is working; and enough wet nappies produced, then the rate of weight gain is unimportant.

Do *not* give complementary feeds. These will reduce the amount of breast milk available because the baby won't want to eat so much and the sucking stimulus is essential for milk production.

Complementary feeds should not be allowed by the mother who wants to breastfeed successfully. As one mother said, 'How can demand and supply work if you suppress half the demand?'

If there is any doubt as to whether your baby is thriving, first increase your milk supply by feeding him more often (see Chapter 10 for details).

Enlightened hospitals have stopped test weighing babies routinely. Test weighing in most cases only worries people unnecessarily: it worries the staff who think a breastfed baby needs the same volume of milk as a bottle-fed baby and it worries the mother because she automatically doubts her ability to feed her baby. Test weighing should be reserved for those babies who are obviously not thriving.

We haven't talked so far about the mother who has her baby at home, mainly because if she has enough help feeding will probably be easier for her. Hospitals are safe places to have babies but they are not ideal when it comes to breastfeeding. Similarly, we haven't mentioned the mother who is discharged home early. Breastfeeding is more successful in both of these groups of mothers – a fact that hospital staff would do well to remember. To try to remedy this state of affairs, some hospitals now have lactation nurses whose sole job is to encourage and advise breastfeeding mothers. With enough help from these specialists, longer stays in hospital need not necessarily militate against successful feeding.

Feeding your baby during these first days in hospital is a somewhat unnatural and often difficult experience. After all, much of hospital ward routine does nothing to help the breastfeeding mother. If you and your baby are well you should be at home in your own environment. All the quiet, loving, constant emotional support and encouragement you need at this time can best be supplied by your family and friends.

8 Feeding day by day

Coping at home

Taking your baby home is an exciting occasion whether or not it's your first. However tempting it is to rush around in hospital making both yourself and the baby look nice for your husband to collect, it's sensible not to overdo it because the last thing you want is to arrive home tired out.

Once you get home, sit down and have a drink and just relax. Leave the washing up, ironing and tidying to someone else for a few days if you possibly can. You'll have your hands quite full enough with the baby. All too often a mother plunges back into her old routine and quickly becomes exhausted. Then when her milk dwindles she's surprised and upset and a vicious circle is set up. For the next few weeks you should relax, eat a nourishing diet and let the world go by as much as possible.

If you have your baby at home or if you are discharged early from hospital, this advice is doubly important. It's unlikely that you would even be allowed to contemplate having a home delivery or an early discharge if your doctor were not sure you had enough help in the home.

Of course, not every baby is a first baby and you may have other children to look after. Hopefully, you and your husband will have made some arrangements with a relative, friend or paid help to come and help out in the first few weeks. Some husbands arrange time off to be at home. Your mother may be the best person to help but nowadays mothers are often not close at hand. Needless to say, if your mother is anti-breastfeeding you'll have to handle the situation especially carefully if you're going to succeed.

A helper or 'doula', as she is called, is a very important member of society in many parts of the world where successful breastfeeding is widely practised. Besides giving practical help a good doula provides emotional support in the first crucial days. Her very presence in the home makes things easier for new mothers because on-the-spot reassurance from someone sympathetic is a godsend. Traditionally a doula is female.

Whatever sort of help you think you'll need, discuss it with your helper before the baby is born so that you both know where you stand. A problem may crop up if the helper wants to look after the baby and expects you to look after the house and other children. Clear this matter up as tactfully and quickly as possible. It's worth deciding whether you are going to feed the baby in front of her or not and such things are easier to decide before the time comes, to avoid hurting anyone's feelings.

How long should your helper stay? This is an individual decision but remember that your milk supply may take several weeks to become properly established and you'll need time to recover from the physical effort of pregnancy and labour. So don't rush her departure, especially if you have more than one child. Make the most of any willing help there may be.

Where to feed

Although in theory you can feed your baby anywhere, you'll find it more pleasurable if you are comfortable. If you find you like cushions to support your arm or the baby, make sure they are left in the chair you use. Having said this, though, there's absolutely no need to make a big thing about certain numbers of cushions, chair height and so on. One woman told us that she stopped breastfeeding because she couldn't bear all the fiddling with cushions! Many mothers find it most relaxing and enjoyable to feed their babies when lying down on a bed or a settee.

If your baby is a winter baby, keep the room warm. Cold air can make the muscle fibres in the areolae and nipples contract and so delay the release of milk. This may frustrate the baby early in a feed. In practice, the warmth of the baby's mouth will warm the nipples and the let-down reflex will make the skin of the breasts feel warm.

If you find you like something to do while you're feeding (and if you haven't got a toddler), keep a book by your chair. One mother we know found a music stand invaluable for holding her book, so leaving her hands free. You may find it relaxing to watch the television or to listen to the radio, though many mothers are quite happy just to watch their baby feeding, especially if he stares up at them as so many babies do. A lot will depend on how long the feed takes – if your baby is a quick feeder, you won't get bored. Feeding should be a time you look forward to and enjoy: if you take care of your own creature comforts, you'll relax, the baby will get the milk easily and everything should go well. In fact, many nursing mothers look forward to feed times as oases of peace in their day. Some babies like quiet feed times and refuse to nurse well in noisy surroundings. Others, particularly older babies, are very easily distracted by other people.

If, on the other hand, you perch on a hard chair to feed, with shoulders aching from supporting the baby's weight and dreading the thought of up to an hour's stint with nothing to do other than look at the baby, it's unlikely that you'll relax, the milk won't let down and your baby will go hungry.

You'll soon find that it's quite possible to feed your baby as you walk around. This means that you can fetch something you want or answer the telephone in the middle of a feed without disturbing your baby.

Many mothers find they get very thirsty when feeding, especially in the first few weeks. If you do, get yourself something to drink before you start so as to avoid interrupting the feed.

Where to keep the baby during the day

If you put your baby in his room to sleep during the day, you run the risk of not hearing when he wakes. Try keeping him sleeping in a carrycot in the room where you are or at least well within earshot. That way you'll know when he wakes and will be able to nurse him as soon as he cries. Household noise is unlikely to keep him awake if he really wants to sleep, and if he doesn't it'll be more interesting for him to watch and listen to what's going on than to lie in a quiet room gazing at the ceiling. Having said this, you don't have to put your baby in a cot between feeds. Many babies are most content when they are carried around in a baby sling or in their mother's arms for most of the day.

How often will feeds be? (see also pages 15 and 86)

Our experience tells us that more misleading advice has been given about this than about anything else to do with breastfeeding and that this advice has done a lot of harm to breastfeeding over the past fifty years or more.

Your baby is unlike any other baby – he's an individual and not just a stomach to be filled every three or four hours by the clock. His only way of telling you he is hungry is by fidgeting or crying, given that in the West we don't carry our babies by our naked breasts so that they can feed when they want without even asking. Some mothers swear they can separate their baby's cries into hunger cries, wet and dirty cries, bored cries and so on. We think that this is unlikely in the first few weeks, when all cries sound pretty much the same to the new mother or anyone else. The only way to decide whether his cry is a 'hungry' one is to offer him the breast. As young babies prefer to have frequent small feeds, he'll almost certainly drink. This is what is known as feeding on demand – *any cry should be interpreted as a request for food until proven otherwise*. There may be the odd occasion when he is clearly not interested in feeding but almost every time he will be. When he's content, then change his nappy if necessary.

Don't be misled by all the advice you are bound to be given by friends, relatives, professionals, baby feeding pamphlets from cows' milk formula manufacturers and old-fashioned baby books. Many of these sources of information include the old chestnuts about feeding the baby every four hours (two a.m., six a.m., ten a.m., two p.m., six p.m. and ten p.m.). This advice is for the birds and bottle-fed babies, not for you and your baby! A few women produce enough milk with such a routine but most find their milk supply slowly dwindles simply because six feeds a day don't give the breasts enough stimulation in these vital early weeks.

Once you accept that your baby may ask for feeds very erratically you're halfway towards feeding successfully. If you worry each time he wants the breast soon after being fed, you're on the path to losing your milk, as worry tends to prevent the let-down reflex from working.

During these early weeks you may find you seem to be spending a large part of the day feeding your baby. That may be but it's worth accepting and enjoying it and not resenting it. Babyhood doesn't go on for long. Don't forget that your baby may want much more frequent feeds if he is unwell or upset.

Although many babies establish a routine after a time, not all do, so don't compare your baby with any other. As we've said already, the baby who wants frequent feeds will stimulate his mother's breasts and hence her milk supply better than the baby who asks for only five or six feeds a day. If in fact your baby asks only for five feeds a day, be very wary and try giving him more, as five episodes of suckling are not really enough to keep up the milk supply in most women. One researcher has noticed that cutting the number of feeds down to five a day leads to an insufficiency of milk in one out of three women. We have found that many successfully breastfeeding mothers cannot say how many feeds they give their baby in a day.

How long will feeds be? (see also pages 17 and 88)
Again, let your baby tell you. The old rule of ten minutes a side was created because that was the average length of time babies needed for a bottle feed. Not all babies are average, though, so whereas some of them will need much less than ten minutes a side, some will want much more. During the first few months you may find that your baby has periods when he wants to feed (or at least to be at the breast) almost continuously for several hours. This is not unusual and is his way of increasing your milk supply. People will tell you that a baby gets most of the milk he needs in the first few minutes at each breast. There is an element of truth in this but studies have shown that not *all* babies get what they need as quickly. Every baby is different. A lot will depend on how vigorously your baby sucks, the strength of your let-down reflex and the time taken for the let-down to start working. Some babies like to play at the breast and feed sporadically while others go for speed above all else.

Another factor to bear in mind is that some babies enjoy sucking even if they have emptied the breast. This can be pleasant for you too and there is no reason to stop unless you want to do something else or have any soreness of the nipples. This *comfort sucking* is thought by many psychologists to be an important factor in the baby's emotional development. The dummy or thumb is the bottle-fed baby's substitute for comfort suckling at the breast. All the time your baby is sucking for comfort he is also stimulating your breasts to make more milk.

Among the primates, the young suck whenever possible and by no means always because of hunger. Human infants are no different. The main reason for the small number of short breast-feeds many babies have in the West each day is the relative inaccessibility of the breast and the reluctance of some mothers to offer it (because of cultural attitudes) for comfort. The large number of mothers whose milk dries up have invariably allowed their baby to suck only if he is 'certifiably' hungry. Babies don't like to suck only for food, fluid and comfort. They may also just enjoy being at the breast when they are happy, or even when they're bored.

As your baby gets older, he'll finish his feeds more quickly unless he's tired, bored, ill or upset.

So what's the answer? There isn't one. When your baby seems to have finished one side – when he becomes less interested in feeding – change him to the other side and let him carry on there as long as he wants to or for as long as you can. *Don't watch the clock*. Primitive peoples don't have clocks and they feed their babies more success-fully than we do!

One breast or two?

Many babies drink from only one breast during a feed. Provided you alternate the breast you give at each feed and the baby is satisfied, this is fine. Giving both breasts at each feed is a western idea and is often not done in those parts of the world where breastfeeding is done more naturally and schedules are unknown. If your baby is extra hungry or fussy, give him both breasts, perhaps even changing sides several times during a feed. One breast at a time fits in well with the baby who wants frequent small feeds, as many prefer. (See also page 175.)

Your baby's feeding pattern and behaviour (see also page 235)

Though each baby is unique as far as his appetite, demand for the breast, sucking pattern and behaviour at the breast go, experienced observers can group breastfeeding babies into several categories. Which category your baby falls into will depend on his personality, his past experience at the breast, how hungry he is and on the way your milk is let down. Some babies always take a long time over feeds and enjoy spending what seems like all day (and night) at the breast, sucking on and off. Once you're sure that your baby is thriving (plenty of wet nappies and putting on weight), then you can stop a feeding session after half an hour or so if you want to do something else. Most of the time, though, try to relax and enjoy this special time with your young baby. Sooner or later he'll start to take his milk more quickly and may want to spend less time at the breast.

Another group of babies regurgitate several times throughout a feed and afterwards, sometimes bringing up most of the milk they've just drunk. All you can do is have patience and give your baby more milk if he wants it. If all the stimulation from having to repeat feeds makes your milk gush very fast, try expressing some before your baby goes to the breast. (See also page 147.)

Many babies, especially if they are small, jaundiced or affected by the drugs you had during labour, snooze every so often during a feed. Don't make the mistake of thinking that the feed is over the first time your baby snoozes. Just calmly wait and he'll wake up again when he has more energy.

You may have the sort of baby who drinks in a very forthright, no-nonsense manner. Feeds from him are over quickly and his behaviour is much more like that of older babies. You could say he has grown up ahead of his time. Lots of babies behave differently at different times of the day and many change their feeding behaviour as they grow older.

Night feeds

The easiest and most natural way of feeding your baby at night is to have him in bed with you all night. This means you'll hardly have to wake up to feed him, because you simply feed him lying down. There'll be no disturbing night-time crying to wake the rest of the household because you can feed him as soon as he becomes restless. And you'll know that he's safe, warm and in the most natural place – next to his mother.

There are no rules about where the baby should be in your bed, but it's easy if you leave your sleeping baby lying by the breast he was at last. When he next wants to be at the breast, roll over with him in your arms close to your chest so that he is lying by your other side by your full breast. Some mothers can manage to feed their baby from the opposite breast by leaning towards him. You'll find that the most comfortable way to lie with your baby is with your arm crooked round the top of his head. This will mean that you can keep one hand on his back to keep him in place at your breast. Once he is old enough to roll over, you may want to put a chair against the side of the bed to stop him rolling out at night. There's usually no need to turn a light on at night unless you have to change a nappy. In the early days your baby may be restless and you may have to sit up with him on your lap for some of the night feeds. You can wind him if necessary simply by holding him in a sitting position while you are lying down. Don't forget to leave something for yourself to drink by your bed. Many mothers feel very thirsty when actually feeding.

You may like to read an interesting book called *The Family Bed* by Tine Thevenin, available from PO Box 16004, Minneapolis, MN 55416, USA. Various aspects of bed sharing are discussed, including the pros and cons.

Many people are horrified at the suggestion that babies should sleep with their parents. Many mothers fear that they'll roll on or suffocate the baby but the chances of doing this are virtually nil. Millions of women the world over sleep with their children quite safely. One of the commonest arguments we hear against this practice is that the baby will become dependent on the mother for sleeping and that he'll be loath to sleep in his own cot or bed when he's older. One way round this is to get him off to sleep in his bed at bedtime by lying down with him to feed him. This can mean that there'll be a period during which he'll be first in his bed and then in yours when he wakes up and needs feeding and comforting. Many families go through a transitional phase of 'musical beds' for some months. The youngest child will probably enjoy sleeping with an older brother or sister when he's around two.

Some mothers feel guilty about having their baby in bed with them. They're uneasy at the thought of prolonged physical contact in bed with their child and some even feel it's incestuous if the child is a boy. This is obviously nonsense.

The only people who we suggest should not have their baby in bed are the very obese; those taking sleeping tablets or hard or soft drugs; and those who go to bed drunk (or whose spouse does). For all other couples sleeping with the baby is perfectly safe.

Should you or your husband decide that you don't want to sleep with your baby, make things as easy as you can for yourself at night by keeping the baby's cot near your bed, preferably so close that you don't even have to get out of bed to lift him in when he cries. This often isn't easy as most cots are not the right height but if your husband is a do-it-yourselfer he will be able to modify the cot to bring the level of the mattress nearer to that of your bed. Hopefully, cot manufacturers will start making them so that the drop side can be lowered to the level of a standard bed.

Keep nappies by the bed so that they are to hand. Your baby will probably go to sleep quite happily without a nappy change at all after night feeds. 'One-way' nappy liners will help keep his skin dry.

If you can't sleep with the baby in your room, or don't want to, then either bring him back with you into your bed to feed, where you'll both be warm and comfy, or put on your dressing gown and feed him in his room. If your baby has a single bed in his own room instead of a cot, you can lie by him to feed him. There is less risk of him staying awake if the room is dark.

When will your baby stop having night feeds? This again is very much an individual matter. Research suggests that breastfed babies go on waking at night for longer. Your baby may give up his night feeds early, in which case you must make sure that you breastfeed often enough during the day to keep up your milk supply and stop your breasts becoming engorged. You may have to express some milk before you go to bed or even during the night to prevent discomfort. Some mothers wake their babies for a feed before they go to bed if they have given up night feeds too early and the milk supply seems to be dwindling. On the other hand your baby may want to continue with one, two or more night feeds for many months or even longer. If your baby wants feeding more often than once or twice your husband may help by getting up for you and bringing him to you in bed, then putting him back into his cot after the feed. Babies often want frequent feeds when they're very young and occasionally for the odd night or two when they are older, so it's worth accepting and coping with them as best you can. Sleep patterns change, sometimes for the better and sometimes for the worse, but all young children grow up and night waking doesn't last for ever – though it may seem like it at the time! Broken nights will make you tired, so you'll have to try to catch up on your sleep during the day. Your relaxation practice at ante-natal classes may come in useful here. One consolation for the breastfeeding mother is that bottle-fed babies often take much longer to settle after a night feed than do breastfed babies.

Many mothers notice during the first few weeks of breastfeeding particularly that when their breasts are full, they feel hot and may sweat suddenly. This is especially likely to happen at night. It is a helpful signal that the time has come to feed your baby – the longer that full breasts are left unemptied, the more likely they are to become engorged – so wake your baby up.

It'll be easier for you not to wear a bra at all and in the early weeks this will help prevent any soreness of your nipples by letting the air get to the nipple skin.

How to get your baby off to sleep

Don't make the mistake of thinking that your new baby will necessarily spend most of the time between feeds asleep, as many baby books would have you believe. Each baby is an individual and will have his own sleep requirements. These will change from day to day according to how he feels and what you've been doing with him, and will also change as he grows older. In general, young babies sleep as much as they need, unlike some older children who sometimes seem to get more and more tired and can't or won't go to sleep. While some babies go straight off to sleep with a full tummy after a feed, others choose this time to stare at their mothers, to look around and, later, to smile and coo. Don't waste such a valuable time for getting to know and love your baby by trying to get him off to sleep if he's not ready.

You'll be told – especially by the older generation, many of whom were slaves to routine – to put your baby in his cot after he's been fed and winded. If he doesn't go off to sleep, the advice is usually to let him cry until he does. Sometimes a time limit on the crying makes it seem less inhumane. *We think that a baby should never be left to cry himself to sleep.* Crying tells you he's unhappy, so it's better to find another way of helping him to go to sleep peacefully and happily. The easiest way of doing this is to let him stay at the breast until he goes to sleep. Most new babies will fall asleep at the breast eventually. If you want to bring up a bubble of wind, do so and then put the baby back to the breast. Some babies doze at the breast at the end of a feed, waking up every so often to nibble or lightly suck at the breast, but never actually letting go. If you gently remove your breast, you may find that your baby drifts into a deeper sleep. If you watch him now, you'll notice that he makes occasional sucking or mouthing movements as though he were still at the breast and, from time to time, a smile or a frown will flicker across his face as he dreams. Similar facial movements can often be seen just before waking. Once your baby is sound asleep and you've had enough time to enjoy cuddling him, put him somewhere warm, safe and within earshot to sleep.

Some babies drop off to sleep regularly in the car, pram or sling, lulled by the motion or noise. Rocking your baby in your arms is another way of inducing sleep in a tired baby who no longer wants to suck at the breast.

Other babies happily go to sleep after a feed if put in a warm, comfortable, familiar place near their mothers.

You'll find that how you get your baby off to sleep will vary with the time of day, where you are and what you're doing. Though many babies prefer to go to sleep in a familiar place, especially when they're older, just you being there feeding him, simply cuddling him on your lap, or lying down by him is enough to reassure most babies as they drop off. There's nothing more pleasant than going to sleep yourself with your baby by you. If you can find the time to nap with your baby, you'll wake up feeling refreshed. You may find he sleeps extra well when you're there, perhaps because of the familiar and reassuring smell, feel and sound of your body. Lots of babies open their eyes several times as they go off to sleep as if to check that their mother is still there.

Your baby may fall into a pattern of sleeping for a certain length of time between some feeds, or he may be a a very irregular sleeper. Lots of young babies wake up very soon after what you thought was the end of a feed and want to go back to the breast. This is quite normal behaviour and is not 'bad'. As long as you haven't pinned your hopes on having an hour or two free, it doesn't matter at all. Simply put the baby back to your breast. Carrying an unsettled baby in a sling is often the answer when you have to get on with essential jobs. It's easier to cook, clean, wash up, write and so on with the baby slung on your back rather than on your front.

Leaking

The leaking you'll have noticed during the first few weeks will gradually become less of a problem. This is partly because the let-down reflex becomes more controlled as your milk supply is established and partly because the storage capacity of the milk ducts increases during the first few weeks so that they can hold more of the let-down milk without allowing it to escape. You'll still notice leaking from the opposite breast during a feed.

How you'll feel throughout the day

As milk is secreted constantly by the milk-producing cells of the breasts, the amount of milk in the breast will depend to some extent on the length of time since the last feed. If your baby doesn't wake and your breasts are uncomfortably full, either express some milk or wake him up – after all, *you need him* sometimes to relieve you as much as he needs you at other times to relieve his hunger.

As your baby will hopefully have his longest break between feeds at night, you'll notice this fullness in your breasts first thing in the morning especially. You may even wake up with your nightie and sheets drenched with milk. The early morning feed is often the most pleasant simply because of the very real sense of relief you feel.

During the day the enjoyment you get from feeding will depend to some extent on how busy you are. If feeds are slotted into a packed day, you may not feel very calm and the baby may sense your tension and be more fussy than usual. Be careful not to be so tense that your let-down doesn't work. If you don't experience the telltale signs (see page 13) then do your best to slow down a bit for the rest of the day and cut out a few jobs the next day. Many mothers feel at their worst in the early evening. Not only do they have to feed the other children and start getting them to bed but they may also want to tidy up the house, feed the baby, and start thinking about supper. The early evening is physiologically a low time for many people anyway. It may all be just too much for you and your let-down reflex so try to organise things so they don't all happen at once. Be your own time and motion expert. Your husband's supper can wait, as long as he understands why and has something to eat to keep him going in the meantime; the other children may be coaxed to clear up their own toys; and you could give them their tea and bath earlier. Do anything to avoid having lots of things to do at the very time of the day when you're beginning to feel tired anyway. Prepare food for the evening in the afternoon, make full use of your refrigerator and freezer and do dishes like casseroles that can be prepared in advance.

Crying baby

The sound of your baby's cry is designed to alert you so that you care for him. It's not the sort of sound that can easily be ignored, even by a stranger, and a baby that won't stop crying is very disturbing. If a baby seems to do nothing but cry for the first few days, weeks or even months, it's hardly surprising that his mother feels something must be wrong with him or his food. Once she is reassured by the doctor that nothing is wrong with the baby, the next stop is often to change the food, and for a breastfeeding mother this means giving the baby a bottle of cows' milk formula.

Is this necessary? In almost every case the answer is no. The first thing to do is to breastfeed, in the way nature intended, which means at least every time the baby cries (see pages 15 and 86). A baby breastfed on schedule will almost certainly cry a lot because not only is he hungry before the clock says it is time for his next feed but he is also denied comfort suckling time because his mother thinks she must allow him only ten minutes on each breast. Feeding a baby when he cries, for as long as he wants to feed, will almost certainly reduce the amount of crying he does. It will also increase your milk supply, which is a good thing if he was crying because he was hungry most of the time. Research has shown that breastfed babies fed on demand cry *much less* than schedule-breastfed babies. It's difficult to find out what the long-term psychological effects of long periods of crying are but they certainly cause unhappiness at the time.

Some babies crave company and settle only when they are held. One way to cope with this if there are things you have to do is to buy a baby sling. There are several on the market which will leave your hands free to get on with your work but which will keep the baby secure and contented next to you as you walk around.

Other babies can be pacified (as long as they are not hungry) by a ride in their pram or in a car. Anything is worth trying but *always try suckling first*.

If all else fails, ask a relative or neighbour to look after the baby for a time. If you are constantly worried about the crying, your milk supply will dwindle and that will make your baby cry more. A change of face and scene often quietens a baby miraculously. If your baby's crying is getting you down emotionally, try to get a break from time to time. If you feel you can't cope any more, tell your health visitor or doctor urgently.

Baby's bowels

A totally breastfed baby's motions are not foul-smelling like those of a bottle-fed baby. They are liquid and passed very frequently at first but later may be passed only every few days. Their normal colour is a bright yellow but occasionally they go green. Often your baby will open his bowels during a feed, so you'll find it saves washing if you change his nappy after a feed, unless he is one of those babies who won't feed in a wet nappy.

Some everyday 'problems'

The mother in a house on her own will come up against some practical problems when she is feeding her baby. For instance, what does she do if the doorbell rings? There are several ways round this. You can decide that when you are feeding, nothing is going to stop you, so you don't answer the bell. You can do up your clothes quickly and answer the door either with your hungry baby crying in your arms or left safely somewhere. You can carry on feeding and answer the door anyway, perhaps with a shawl round you. Or you can make a little notice for the front door which says, 'I am feeding my baby. Only ring if it is important, please.'

What about the window cleaner? That's easier. Keep a nappy or shawl near you when you are feeding so that you can do a cover-up job to preserve your modesty and spare his embarrassment! Practise first so that you learn how to do it without annoying the baby.

The telephone is more difficult because somehow it always seems such an urgent noise and it's difficult to steel yourself to leave it unanswered. One way round this is to take the phone off the hook while you're feeding. Another is to have the phone by you. This may need organising with the telephone company who can put the phone anywhere you want provided you pay for the alteration.

With any of these disturbances, what you don't want to happen is for your let-down to be inhibited and for the feed to be spoilt, so it's worth thinking about how you are going to cope before you actually have to. Your let-down will work best when you are calm and undisturbed.

Feeding with children around

A new baby in the family is both a joy and a misery to the other children, especially if they are very young themselves. The attractions of the new acquisition are tempered by the fact that mother now has a new central interest in her life which seems to take up much of her time.

The way round this is to be extra loving, especially to your youngest child, because it is probably he who will be most affected by the new baby. If he wants to have a feed, let him – he's only trying to compete for your attention and will soon get fed up with the breast. Some mothers carry on breastfeeding throughout pregnancy and then feed the older child and the baby, which tends to reduce jealousy.

Always try to bring your older child into the breastfeeding circle. Soon you'll be so adept at breastfeeding that you'll be able to sit reading to a toddler and feeding the baby at the same time. If you find you can't do this then keep an absorbing toy or game handy for when you're feeding or reserve a few minutes to play alone later with the child who feels left out.

How to feed in company

Again, there are many ways of coping with this and what you decide to do will depend on you and your feelings of modesty and on the other people involved. You may discover that you always prefer to feed alone, in which case you'll miss hours of other people's company. If you do decide on this, then you can either send visitors into another room when you feed in the room you usually use or you can go into another room yourself. You and the baby are just as important as the visitors. Don't hurry the feed in order to get back to your friends and show off the baby. The baby will be much more likely to be in a good mood for being shown off if he's well fed and happy and that means feeding him as you normally would.

If you are in someone else's house, make yourself warm and comfortable before you feed and ask for drinks or cushions or whatever you need.

If you are happy to feed in company you might like a few tips.

Some people are embarrassed about seeing a baby being breastfed simply because they are not used to it. If you sense this, your let-down might not work. You can get round this either by sitting at one end of a room so that you can join in the discussion but not be too boldly in evidence, by draping yourself with a shawl to cover both breast and baby or, preferably, by wearing clothes that reveal nothing when you are breastfeeding. Of course some people are delighted to see a baby fed naturally and are not at all embarrassed.

A clever choice of clothing is also useful for when you are in a train, bus, park or eating out – all occasions when other people may be embarrassed even if you're not. If you pull up a T-shirt, jumper or blouse from the waist you can feed very discreetly and show nearly nothing at all. Clothes that unbutton are more revealing. A practice feed in front of a mirror may give you confidence.

Entertaining

If looking after people and cooking for them comes easily to you, then you'll probably find breastfeeding no hindrance to entertaining. However, if you're the sort of person who worries for days about what to give friends to eat, then think twice about entertaining. It's as simple as that. Whatever you cook, make sure it's something that won't be harmed by being left in a warm oven if you have to feed the baby before you eat. The calmer you are, the calmer the baby will be as babies quickly pick up their mother's feelings and react to them. It's perfectly possible with a little practice to feed a baby even at the dinner table in a way that will offend no one.

Car journeys and holidays

Breastfeeding is easy in a car – in fact it really comes into its own when you're travelling. Either stop and feed or carry on (with your partner driving, of course!) and feed the baby in the back seat for safety. You should have no problem at all.

If you are going to fly, it's not a bad idea to fly at night so that the baby will be sleepy, the aircraft dark for feeding and the chances of your having more privacy increased because fewer passengers move about. Some airlines have a special seat that can be curtained off for the breastfeeding mother but the most practical answer is to feed discreetly in the main part of the aircraft.

When you're travelling, don't get exhausted. Let your husband do as much as possible or you could impair your let-down reflex temporarily.

Holidays are much simpler with a breastfed baby. There's no cleaning and sterilising to worry about, no boiled water to organise for a feed and the equipment necessary is always to hand.

Going out

Whenever you go out, try to take your baby with you. Once your baby has become used to you being there all the time a bottle (even of breast milk) may not comfort him. What he wants is his mother.

If you *have* to go out without your baby you can leave a bottle of your own expressed milk. Expressed milk can be left in the fridge in a sterile bottle and the bottle warmed up in a bowl of hot water when needed by your babysitter. If the baby is hungry enough he'll drink from the bottle and because the milk is his usual brew, there should be no fuss. If he's reluctant to drink from the bottle, then leave instructions with your sitter to give the milk from a sterilised spoon.

We have already described the technique of expressing milk (see page 94). The difficulty is collecting enough. Try expressing after every feed for two days before you are due to go out. In this way you should get enough milk to satisfy your baby if you go out for an evening. The milk can be expressed directly into a bottle and kept in the fridge for up to three days. You'll notice that the milk goes into layers on standing but these soon disappear when it is warmed.

It's obviously easier to take the baby with you wherever you go and apart from going to the theatre, cinema, a restaurant or a few other places, it should almost always be possible.

If you and your husband go out to friends for the evening, then take the baby with you, even if you have a sitter for the older children. If the baby wants feeding, it's a simple enough matter to pop upstairs and feed (if by staying you'd offend the other guests). If your hostess has been warned in advance that you are bringing your breastfed baby, she won't have cooked anything that might spoil if left in the oven for a little longer.

Feeding a baby from day to day is one of the most rewarding things in a woman's life, yet may not be as easy as she thinks. Knowing what to do is half the battle. Knowing what can go wrong is the other.

9 Looking after yourself

Why?

There are two very good reasons for looking after yourself when you've had a baby. Firstly, as wife and mother you're probably the kingpin of your home and if you are well and happy the chances are that the rest of the family will be happy too. If, like so many mothers, you get tired and run down with the pressures of house, husband, other children and a baby to look after, then your mood will reflect on the other people in the house.

Secondly, a fit and healthy mother is far more likely to breastfeed her baby successfully than the mother who is permanently physically and emotionally exhausted. This is not so much because the amount of milk produced will be greater – we don't know whether this is so or not – or the quality of the milk will be different, but is because an exhausted mother's let-down reflex just won't be as reliable. Once the let-down reflex becomes unreliable, the baby gets frustrated at each feed and is likely to take less and less milk, become hungry, cry more and so add to the mother's exhaustion.

As we've already described, 'mothering the mother' is seen as a vital part of successful child-rearing in many cultures. These wise people know that a well-cared-for mother stands more chance of rearing her young children happily. In our culture, it's unlikely that you will have somebody to look after you all the time, even if you manage to arrange for a helper to come in for part of the day, so you must make sure that you look after yourself and make this one of your priorities for everyone's sake.

Rest, relaxation and sleep

If you have only one baby, you'll find it comparatively easy to make time for catnaps during the day when he sleeps. Indeed, if you are waking up several times a night, which is highly likely, especially at first, you *must* make time for naps, even if you are the sort of person who would have turned her nose up at daytime sleeping before you had the baby.

For the mother who comes home after forty-eight hours in hospital, rest – and that means rest in bed – is *not* a luxury, it's a must. It's a pretty safe rule to say that you should aim to be spending most of your day in and around your bed for the first week after the birth whether you're in hospital or at home. This doesn't mean you should stay in bed *all day* – you shouldn't. But you certainly shouldn't be busying yourself around the house.

The temptation, especially for the efficient sort of woman who held down a busy job before she had her baby, is to cram all sorts of household and other tasks into the baby's sleep time. As we've said before, you have the rest of your life to be a superwoman – you don't have to be one now. If you can be rested, cheerful and happy, you'll be a far better mother than if you'd cleaned the oven, changed the sheets, written ten letters and exhausted yourself! Keep your kitchen and bathroom clean, pick up obvious fluff and tidy up things left lying around – that's all you need to do to keep your home pleasant. Housework is always there but you'll probably have a chance to mother a new baby only a couple of times in a lifetime, so make the most of them.

Whenever you can, then, relax. Even if you don't sleep during the day, lie down and read or put the radio on. Think about moving the TV into the bedroom. Use your relaxation training from ante-natal classes to get rid of unnecessary tension. You can even do this when you're feeding the baby, peeling the vegetables, watching television or driving the car. The secret is not to let undue muscle tension build up.

Breastfeeding naturally, with no schedules, helps ensure that newly delivered mothers sit down quietly for long periods.

At night you'll just need to accept that it'll probably be a long time before you regularly have a long, unbroken stretch of sleep. If you go back to sleep quickly when you've fed the baby, so much the better. If you can't, don't worry, just relax. At least you'll be getting physical rest. If you keep your baby in bed with you, you'll be able to snooze during feeds.

The mother with more than one child has a much harder task if she is to get enough rest. If the elder child still sleeps during the day, then she should try to get the baby to sleep as well so she can have a rest at the same time. If this is impossible, then it's a good idea to lie down anyway with your baby – that's always more relaxing than sitting in a chair. Sometimes you'll be able to get a neighbour or a friend to help by taking the toddler off your hands for an hour while you sleep. He'll probably like the change too. An extension of this is to get a group of local mothers together so that you can help each other out.

Your food

There is no evidence that any food, drink or vitamins will increase or decrease your milk supply (see Chapter 10) *provided you eat an adequate, well-balanced, nutritious diet.* It's sensible to eat according to your appetite and not to try to lose weight – the fat stores you have accumulated during pregnancy will slowly be lost with breast-feeding as long as you are not overeating. The mother who eats sensibly not only provides her baby with plenty of milk but also makes sure that her own body isn't drained of food resources for the baby's sake.

Even severely malnourished mothers in developing countries manage to feed their babies for three months before extra food is necessary for the normal growth of the baby. However, they often do this at the expense of their own bodies – they can become short of calcium and protein, for example. The more babies these women have and feed, the poorer their physical state becomes. We must stress, though, that this situation is virtually never seen in the affluent West where almost everyone has enough to eat.

What would happen if you didn't eat enough? There's a chance that you might not produce as much milk as you could and that your baby might go hungry. The actual quality of your milk is said to be relatively little affected. Obviously you can't go on a slimming spree while you're feeding.

How much extra should you eat? This is a vexed question that experts have been discussing for years. Recommended extra calorie allowances change every few years in the light of more up-to-date knowledge. What we can say, though, is that you should eat slightly more than you do when you are not pregnant or breastfeeding (that is, if you usually eat normally and manage to keep your weight steady). Given that the baby under six months needs an average (depending on size) of between 600 and 800 calories daily from you and given that your accumulated fat stores built up during pregnancy should supply 300 calories daily to the milk, then it would seem that you should be eating an extra 300 to 500 calories a day. Some experts have found that mothers breastfeeding successfully eat on average almost 700 calories a day more than bottle-feeding mothers and still manage to lose weight.

There have been suggestions from research work that the milk supply is more dependable if the mother's calorie intake is evenly spaced throughout the day, rather than the bulk being eaten at one meal.

Is there anything you should eat more of when you are feeding your baby? No. Assuming you're eating a good diet, just eat slightly more of everything and you'll be all right.

Provided your diet is well-balanced, there's absolutely no need to drink a lot of milk. Indeed, if you don't like milk there's no need to drink any at all! Cows' milk doesn't make breast milk. Cows don't drink milk but manage to make plenty of milk from their diet of grass. No mammal needs milk to make milk. Some sources of dietary information for pregnant and nursing mothers recommend that lots of milk (one to two pints daily) should be drunk. In the light of what is known about allergy today, most experts consider it unwise for a pregnant or nursing mother to eat or drink a large amount of any one food, especially if there is a family history of allergic disorders. As cows' milk is so common an allergen, a large intake is best avoided both during pregnancy and while feeding. It's sensible to see cows' milk in perspective. It's not a magic food but simply one of many foods that we can choose to include in our daily diet. Its advantages are that it is relatively cheap and that it contains a wide range of nutrients. All of these can, however, be absorbed from many other foods besides dairy foods provided you eat a balanced diet (see page 77).

Some spicy foods like garlic and curry can come through in the milk but as far as we know they have no effect on the baby. The vast majority of foods seem to have little affect even though traces may get through into the milk. There are no foods that are absolutely forbidden, but should you find that your baby reacts in an unusual way to your breast milk after you have eaten a certain food, then cut it out while you're breastfeeding. Some babies are certainly more sensitive to the foods their mothers eat than others. Onions and cabbage are two foods reported by some mothers to cause fussing in their babies. Chocolate gives some babies a rash, diarrhoea or constipation and can make them irritable.

You'll find that you are more thirsty than usual and this is scarcely surprising when you consider that the baby will be taking on average between 600 and 800 ml (more than a pint) of milk a day from you, depending on the individual baby, his age and weight. There is no need to force yourself to drink more – just drink as much as you want to. Research has shown that drinking more than your thirst demands actually reduces the amount of milk you produce.

Many nursing mothers feel most thirsty while they are actually feeding, so keep something by you then if this applies to you.

Many mothers worry whether or not they should drink anything alcoholic. Drinking in moderation is acceptable. Some alcohol will pass into your breast milk and if you drink large amounts, correspondingly more will get to the baby. Some babies are temporarily uncomfortable and irritable after their mother has had a drink and the type of drink seems to be important. There is a report of an eight-day-old baby who became drunk after the mother had had 750 ml (well over a pint) of port in a period of twenty-four hours! Drinking enough to make you feel 'tipsy' may harm your milk supply by affecting your oxytocin output and so making your let-down reflex unreliable, so go easy! (See page 200.)

The caffeine from a moderate intake (more than six to eight cups) of tea, coffee or other caffeine-containing drinks can accumulate in a breastfed baby and cause abnormal activity and sleeplessness which disappears when the mother has been off the caffeine for a few days. Smoking increases the effects of caffeine. If you suspect that you may be drinking too much caffeine, try cutting out tea and coffee for a week to see if this makes any difference to your baby.

Smoking may reduce your milk supply. Nicotine in large amounts has other unpleasant side effects too, so it's a good idea to cut out smoking completely if you can and at any rate to cut down the number of cigarettes you smoke while you're breastfeeding. Heavy smoking (more than twenty to thirty cigarettes a day) may not only decrease your milk supply and interfere with your let-down but may cause nausea and vomiting in your baby. Though your inhaled nicotine gets into your milk, it is not very well absorbed by the baby from his gut into his bloodstream. However, he breathes in large amounts second-hand if you smoke near him (especially if you blow smoke at his face) and this also applies if other people smoke near him. Inhaling cigarette smoke increases his risk of getting respiratory disorders such as pneumonia and bronchitis and also puts him at a greater risk of dying from the sudden infant death syndrome. Researchers have also found that in the milk of mothers who smoke there is more DDT.

Contraception

Unless you don't mind having another baby soon, you'll need to take contraceptive precautions even if you're fully breastfeeding. Although, as we've seen on page 57, you won't ovulate for some time, breastfeeding can't be relied upon as a 100-per-cent safe contraceptive, even if you are feeding on a completely unrestricted basis.

If you decide not to take contraceptive pills (see page 203) this means you will have to use some sort of barrier method or, later, an intra-uterine contraceptive device. Probably the safest and most satisfactory contraceptives to use soon after a baby are diaphragms and sheaths. A diaphragm should be fitted by your doctor and should be used with a spermicidal cream. A sheath for your husband may be the most practical and satisfactory method overall until you stop breastfeeding.

Shopping

If you normally travel some way to the shops you'll find in the early weeks that you will have very little time between feeds to do the shopping. You can get round this by doing a big weekly shop with your husband and the car or by getting the shops to deliver. Some mothers still have corner shops near them. There's nothing worse than going shopping and having to wheel a hungry, crying baby home in a laden pram when you're feeling tired yourself.

Seeing friends

While some women like their own company best, many others feel very lonely if they leave their jobs, have a baby and don't bother to make friends. A baby is a very good conversation opener and you'll probably find it easier to make friends now than at any other time. Breastfeeding is absolutely no hindrance to seeing people –

especially other mothers – during the day. It's best not to arrange set times for meetings at other people's houses because you'll probably end up breaking appointments when your baby wants to spend long, unhurried times at the breast. If you ask friends to your house, remember to look after your baby first and foremost. They can make drinks and answer the front door for you if necessary and will probably enjoy feeling useful.

One last word. Don't expect to get back to feeling like your old self overnight. Having a baby is physically and emotionally very demanding and many women don't feel like their real selves for the first month. Some women say that it takes a full year to get back to normal physically and mentally.

10 Your milk supply

Not enough milk – the commonest problem

Whilst many mothers never have any problems at all with supplying the right amount of milk for their babies, others find that they have too much or too little, especially in the early weeks before their milk supply has become properly established. Too much milk is often a nuisance but rarely stops a mother from breastfeeding. Too little milk, however, is the commonest reason mothers give for stopping breastfeeding or for introducing complementary feeds in the first few weeks.

In 1974 the UK Department of Health recommended that mothers should be encouraged to breastfeed their babies for at least the first two weeks of life, but preferably for four to six months. They also concluded that, for most babies, milk alone is adequate for normal growth and development for the first few months of life.

The Working Party of the Panel of Child Nutrition which wrote the report realised that there was a lack of up-to-date information on infant feeding practices on a national scale. To remedy this, large national surveys were undertaken by the Office of Population Censuses and Surveys (OPCS) in 1975 and 1980, each providing a representative sample of all births during a period of one month in England and Wales.

The surveys showed that breastfeeding became much more popular between 1975 and 1980. Not only did more mothers start off by breastfeeding in 1980, but the ones who started carried on for longer than did their counterparts in 1975: for example by four months, 27 per cent of mothers were still breastfeeding compared with only 13 per cent in 1975.

Breastfeeding at ages up to nine months in England and Wales

	1975 %	1980 %
Birth	51	67
1 week	42	58
2 weeks	35	54
6 weeks	24	42
4 months	13	27
6 months	9	23
9 months	–	12

It's interesting to break down the breastfeeding statistics further to see how many mothers gave their babies nothing but breast milk for the first three months at least, as recommended by the Department of Health in 1980. Many of the 'breastfeeding' mothers above were also giving bottles of cows' milk formula or solids. From their mass of information, the researchers concluded that in 1980, at least 28 per cent of six-week-old babies were receiving breast milk alone, compared with 12 per cent in 1975. As for four-month-old breastfed babies, in 1980 at least 14 per cent were receiving only breast milk, whereas in 1975 only 1 per cent were. Clearly mothers today are more likely to breastfeed completely and for longer than before.

However, it's also clear that a lot of babies are getting both breast and bottle milk. Once that happens, a mother is well on the way to weaning her baby from the breast, because although she can increase her milk supply, it's unlikely that she will. Increasing the milk supply requires expert advice and this is often not available.

It's tempting to believe that the mothers who stopped breast-feeding their babies in the first few months did so because they wanted to, but other figures show that this simply wasn't the case. The vast majority of mothers don't stop breastfeeding by choice but because they can't make their milk last for long enough.

Main reason given by mothers for stopping breastfeeding

	Stopped by 6 weeks	Stopped between 6 weeks and 4 months	Stopped between 4 and 6 months
	%	%	%
Insufficient milk	54	66	38
Painful breasts or nipples	12	4	6
Baby wouldn't suck/ rejected the breast	9	4	11
Inverted nipples	6	–	–
Mother ill	5	9	3
Baby ill	2	3	4
Had breastfed long enough/as long as planned	1	5	25
Breastfeeding too tiring/ taking too long	1	1	1
Domestic reasons	2	1	5
Embarrassment	2	1	–
Baby can't be fed by others	1	1	–
Didn't like breastfeeding	2	–	–
Going back to work	–	3	–
Other reasons	3	2	7
	100	100	100

From *Infant Feeding 1975: Attitudes and Practice in England and Wales*, HMSO SS1064.

The message that comes across from this table is that, whatever age the baby was when his mother stopped breastfeeding, by far the most likely reason for her stopping was an insufficiency of milk. This was more important than nipple soreness, far more important than the almost mythical 'going back to work', and beat breastfeeding being 'too tiring' by a long way. The figures for 1980 reflect similar reasons for stopping, with insufficient milk being the most important whatever the age of the baby.

Drying up of milk is the main disorder of breastfeeding in Great Britain, not to mention the rest of the West and, increasingly, the Third World.

The fact that often escapes both mothers and health professionals alike is that an insufficient milk supply is a preventable problem in almost every mother. Just think how much bitter disappointment could be saved if only this were understood.

What advice were these mothers with insufficient milk given before they finally stopped breastfeeding? Amazingly, 94 per cent of them were told by their midwife, health visitor or doctor to give cows' milk formula complements or to stop breastfeeding altogether and to put their babies on the bottle. No mention of increasing the milk supply was made except to the lucky 6 per cent, though such advice should have been given straight away. (Unless, of course, a baby was actually ill because of a lack of breast milk, in which case cows' milk formula or, preferably, donated breastmilk should have been used to supplement the mother's milk while she was encouraged to increase her own milk supply.)

In practice, almost every woman can breastfeed if she wants to and if she is given enough information and help to back her up. It's interesting to note here that all the twenty babies born in one prisoner-of-war camp in Singapore during the Second World War were satisfactorily breastfed for six months before 'supplementary feeding' was started. All the mothers continued to breastfeed until their babies were over a year old.

Experiments in which women who said they hadn't enough milk were given oxytocin injections after a feed showed that in the majority about 50 per cent of the available milk was still in their breasts. Because their milk hadn't been let down adequately (by nature's own oxytocin supply), this 50 per cent was left in the breasts and wasn't available for the baby. Almost every woman can supply about twice the volume of milk her baby needs to thrive. The trouble is that she doesn't always let it down to her baby. Your milk supply *can* be increased – it's simply a question of knowing how.

Is the baby getting enough? (see also page 186)
This is a loaded question – the very fact that it's asked at all is enough to worry many mothers so much that their milk production falls off because their let-down is inhibited and then their babies don't in fact get enough!

It's a question that stems from the years when strict four-hourly schedules were enforced, when many breastfed babies really *didn't* get enough because the schedules didn't allow milk production to reach its full potential.

It's also a question that would rarely need to be asked at all if only mothers were encouraged to breastfeed as nature intended.

However, as so many mothers today are still wrongly advised to restrict suckling time to some sort of schedule or routine, it's a question that must be asked.

If a baby is alert, satisfied after a feed, obviously thriving, if you are giving him at least eight to eleven feeds a day (a typical number), or more, if he can milk the breast well, if you are letting down your milk, and if he has six to eight really wet nappies each day, then he's getting enough. His actual weight gain is not important and there is no need to have him weighed frequently.

In the first month, after any initial weight loss, the *average* weight gain is between four and seven ounces each week; from the second to the fifth month, six to eight ounces a week; from the sixth to the eighth month, four ounces a week; and from the ninth to the twelfth month, two to three ounces a week. Of course, some quite healthy babies regularly put on less than the average and others more. Don't take any notice of your baby's change in weight from one week to another. A healthy, thriving baby sometimes gains no weight or may even lose some in any one week, though the overall rate of gain over the weeks is steady.

If your doctor suggests regular weighing for your baby, the chances are that he'll keep an eye on his rate of weight gain over the weeks as this is a reasonable guide to your baby's progress and health. If he isn't thriving because you're not giving him enough milk or because of some other reason, your doctor will spot this earlier than he otherwise might have done and will hopefully be able to nip the problem in the bud.

If you have your baby weighed regularly, ideally it should be done with nothing on. If he is weighed clothed, make sure that the clothes are similar from week to week.

In general, a baby's expected rate of weight gain can be forecast from his birth weight (though there are exceptions: the weight gain of babies who are extra heavy at birth, compared with average, tends to slow down a little, whereas that of lighter than average babies tends to speed up). If a healthy, full-term baby weighs only a bit more than average, it can be predicted that his rate of weight gain will be more than average, making him heavier than average throughout infancy. Similarly, the rate of gain of a baby weighing a little less than average at birth will be less than average. This method of predicting weight gain has little practical use. Better are the 'percentile' charts which were worked out after studying the weight gain of large numbers of babies. A baby's weight can be plotted on such a chart over a period of time. If a baby's weight gain seems, for example, to be slowing down and leaving his expected 'line' on the chart, then he may be being underfed at the breast or may have a disorder that is preventing him from thriving.

On average, a breastfed baby tends to double his birth weight by four months and triple it by a year.

Whatever you do, don't use any baby scales at home. The neurotic weighing of your baby at home is a sure way to get yourself into a real panic as soon as his weight gain doesn't live up to your perhaps unrealistic expectations. Remember too that the so-called 'normal' weights are often based on bottle-fed (on average over-weight) babies. If your baby consistently lags behind yet is well and happy, don't worry. Research has shown that we are foolish to judge how healthy a baby is by his weight gain in the early months. A study in southern Africa has found that, in communities in which babies gain weight and grow quickly, the population as a whole tends to die younger. Fast early growth goes hand in hand with early senescence.

An underfed baby may cry a lot and not be satisfied after a feed. Also, he won't soak as many nappies as a well-fed one. This is difficult to assess, though, as the nappies of a schedule-fed baby will probably be changed less often so will be quite likely to be very wet anyway. Similarly, an underfed baby will not dirty the nappies as much but this is an unreliable way of deciding whether your baby is getting enough.

Recently doctors have been alarmed by some apparently content and sleepy breastfed babies who are actually starving but are not making their needs known by crying. The reason for these starving babies in the West (where the mothers have enough to eat) is usually that the commonly advised method of feeding three- to five-hourly, ten minutes a side, works only for those few women who have a very plentiful supply of milk. Most of us need to feed our babies much more frequently and for longer periods if we want to build up our milk supply to levels which will satisfy our babies.

If you or your doctor or health visitor thinks that your baby isn't getting enough milk because his weight gain is small or non-existent for a few weeks, don't be put off breastfeeding but take steps straight away to increase your milk supply (see page 138). If complementary feeds are advised, ask for a few days' grace to increase your milk supply first. If you are not confident that you can do this by yourself, ask for the help of your local NCT breastfeeding counsellor or La Leche League leader, who will have helped many mothers with this problem before. She'll reassure you that you can increase your milk supply noticeably within two or three days, and will give you expert guidance on what to do. You'll almost certainly be able to avoid giving complementary cows' milk formula feeds completely. Don't forget that with our society's strange methods of 'token' breastfeeding, even a solely breastfed baby can be underfed, so never be lulled into complacency just because you are breast-feeding but take heed of your doctor's or health visitor's warning and change to a more natural way of breastfeeding (see page 15).

Before we talk about how to increase the milk supply, let's just run through the factors that affect it.

Factors that affect the milk supply
Suckling
We've already seen in Chapter 2 that the more you suckle your baby, the more prolactin is secreted by the pituitary gland, the more milk is produced by the breasts and the better conditioned the let-down reflex becomes. *It's the total length of suckling time each day that is important and that depends on the number and length of the feeds, together with the time given to comfort suckling (see page 109).* Your baby will ask for a certain number of feeds, which you should always give. He may also want to carry on feeding when the milk is finished; you should allow as much of this as you can. You may also have to offer a certain number of unasked-for feeds in order to build up your supply if he's not getting enough.

The let-down reflex
Even if you allow your baby plenty of suckling time, there's a chance that your let-down reflex may not work, in which case the

baby will get only the foremilk. Let-down failure is a very common cause of insufficient milk. The let-down reflex must work if the baby is to get the hindmilk and so empty the breast. If your let-down usually takes two to three minutes to work and you normally restrict suckling time to say ten minutes, your baby will have lost two to three minutes of what you thought was 'drinking time'. While seven to eight minutes' drinking time is enough for some babies, it'll leave others very hungry indeed.

Remember that sometimes your milk may be let down several times during a feed, especially if the baby stays at the breast for a long time. Stopping him before he is ready may mean that he misses out on one of these potential later let-downs.

The degree of emptying of the breast

This is tied up with the last two points. If your baby isn't allowed long enough to empty the breast, if the hindmilk isn't let down at all, or if it is incompletely let down, or if the breast is allowed to remain full for a long period before the baby feeds, then the milk supply will gradually fall off. There are a number of reasons for this. First, the tension in the breast from the build-up of milk reduces the blood supply to the milk glands, so making the milk-producing cells less efficient. Second, the tension actually harms the milk-producing cells, so making them temporarily less able to produce milk. Third, the muscle cells cannot contract so well round the swollen milk glands and so the let-down is less efficient. Whenever your breasts feel full or the slightest bit tense and uncomfortable, you should put your baby to the breast.

Age

Older mothers having their first baby tend to produce less milk at first than do younger ones. This particularly applies to women over thirty. It does not mean that their milk supply cannot be increased.

Attitude

Mothers who *really* want to breastfeed actually produce more milk. One study of mothers' attitudes to feeding their babies found that those who had said they preferred bottle-feeding were three times more likely to say that their baby had refused the breast and twice as likely to say that their baby was a bad feeder when compared with mothers whose intention it was to breastfeed right from the start. Breastfeeding is thus greatly helped by positive attitudes. In the same survey, mothers who wanted to breastfeed reported that their babies refused the bottle!

But, having said this, the fact remains that a lot of women who really want to breastfeed fail because they believe they haven't enough milk. Many a woman's greatest single concern *before* she embarks on breastfeeding is that she won't have enough milk. The worry is ingrained in modern women.

Parity
Mothers having their first babies tend to produce less milk than those who have already had one or more babies. Again, this is not to say that their milk supply cannot be increased.

Diet
Provided you eat well your diet should make no difference to your milk supply, bearing in mind that you should be eating slightly more than normal and drinking according to your thirst. Malnourished women produce less milk, though the quality of their milk is little affected (see also page 124).

The Pill
The contraceptive pill, unless it is of the progestogen-only type, usually reduces the milk supply.

The blood flow through the breast
This is 400 to 500 times the volume of milk produced. The greater the blood flow, the more milk there is.

Bras
Many women wear too tight a bra and then wonder why their milk supply is failing. It is well known that constricting the breasts reduces or even stops the milk supply; in fact this is a well-known method of stopping women lactating. If you have small or medium-sized breasts leave your bra off altogether while you get your milk supply going again and then wear a looser-fitting bra.

How to increase your milk supply

There are two ways of doing this, assuming always that you are eating sensibly. The first is to increase suckling time, that is the number and length of feeds, and the second is to condition the let-down reflex, if this is at fault.

Suckling time

Breastfeeding as commonly practised in the West today is really a sort of token effort. It is governed by schedules and the restriction of suckling time and usually lasts for only a few weeks, during which time cows' milk formula, juices or solids are added to the baby's diet.

Natural breastfeeding depends on the demand and supply principle, which ensures that the breasts automatically produce enough milk for the individual baby. There is no limitation of suckling time and no need for any food supplements for the first three to six months at least.

The first thing to do when increasing suckling time is to *feed your baby when he is hungry*. How do you know when he is hungry? The answer, usually, is when he cries.

You may already be feeding your baby when he cries and yet still not have enough milk for him, in which case there are two things you can do. First, let your baby feed as long as he wants at each breast. Though the average baby may take all the milk he needs in ten minutes at each breast, many babies need very much longer and many a confidently breastfeeding mother reports that her baby sometimes likes to stay at the breast for up to an hour or even as long as two or three hours, especially in the early evening, suckling much of the time and letting go for a few minutes' nap every so often. This is something the baby books and pamphlets don't tell the inexperienced breastfeeding mother, so when her baby shows signs of wanting a long feeding session, she panics and thinks that something is wrong. Nothing is wrong with a baby wanting to stay at the breast. He's just behaving normally. If he's thriving, you can curtail his feeds if you haven't the time or inclination to sit with him. However, if you're trying to increase your milk supply, try to take a positive pleasure in keeping your baby at the breast when he wants to, because this is a good way of increasing your nipples' stimulation and hence your milk supply. No harm will come from occasionally cutting a feed short, for instance if you have to pick up older children from school but, as a general rule, let your baby stop only when he wants to.

Second, fit in some extra feeds, perhaps even twice as many, even if your baby doesn't actually ask for them. This may mean waking him up but, as it's for his own good (and yours), do it anyway. Try not to let more than two hours elapse between the beginning of one feed and the beginning of the next, except perhaps when you are in bed.

If you increase your baby's suckling time by building up the number *and* length of his feeds, then your milk supply will improve because of the greater secretion of prolactin, the conditioning of the let-down reflex and the better and more frequent emptying of the breasts. This usually takes at least two to three days.

It may be a help to a mother trying to increase her milk supply if she stops thinking of the time her baby spends at her breast as a *feed*. Though babies of course get all their food from the breast, they also get comfort and pleasure from being there. What's more, the movements of their tongue, cheek and jaw muscles are stimulating optimal development of these areas. Instead of thinking of time at the breast as a time when you are trying to get as much milk into your baby as quickly as possible, calm down and consider it as a time when your baby is doing his own thing. Babies grow up quickly and the time will come soon enough when your child wants to be independent. Enjoy his loving dependency while you can. It's interesting that members of one African tribe were flummoxed when asked by researchers about their breastfed babies' feeding times. They apparently didn't equate the times their babies spent at the breast with them getting food at all! They simply put their babies to the breast because that seemed to be what the babies wanted to make them happy.

Some babies themselves diminish their mother's milk supply by sucking their thumbs or fingers instead of wanting to breastfeed. These babies have often been denied comfort sucking time at the breast in the past. A dummy can have the same effect and should be discarded if the milk supply is to be increased.

Giving solids or drinks of juice or water can reduce a baby's demand for the breast. Breast milk is much more important than any of these additions in the first few months, so don't hesitate to cut them out if they are interfering with your baby's need to breast-feed.

Occasionally, the milk supply can diminish simply because the baby is lulled by being continually carried in a baby sling or carrier, or on a hip, and just doesn't ask for feeds. To remedy this, put the baby to the breast much more often than he seems to want.

Going back to work often coincides with a decrease in milk production. Put your baby to the breast as much as he wants when you are at home and express your milk frequently at work to increase your milk supply (see page 151).

The let-down reflex

As we explained in Chapter 2, the let-down reflex is readily influenced by such factors as fatigue, anxiety, fear and pain, so much so that these factors can completely prevent the let-down of milk. During the first few weeks or months the let-down is more vulnerable than later when the milk supply has become established and the nursing mother is more confident in her ability to feed her baby. This goes part of the way towards explaining why a mother nursing her second baby is more successful from the start than when she nursed her first.

When we talk of the establishment of the milk supply, we mean that the let-down reflex has become so well conditioned through practice that it virtually never fails and also that the mother's breasts are matching their milk supply to the baby's demands, with no surplus or shortage.

A poor milk supply due to an unreliable let-down reflex is one of the commonest problems of breastfeeding but, once you understand what is happening, there's every chance of putting it right. Successful breastfeeding depends as much on good drainage of the milk that is produced (which of course depends on the proper working of the let-down reflex) as on the actual amount that is produced.

One useful trick when increasing your milk supply is to try 'switch nursing'. Feed your baby first at one breast, then at the other, then start all over again. If you're feeding your baby two hourly, you might like to give him ten minutes at each breast each time, which will mean you're feeding him for about forty minutes every two hours. The time taken is a small price to pay for an increase in your milk supply.

How do you know if the let-down reflex is working?

In the early days you'll know by the afterpains in the womb early in a feed and by a tingling feeling in the breasts together with spraying or leaking of milk from the nipples. The skin of the breasts feels warmer than usual and any initial nipple pain disappears as the milk floods through, so equalising the negative pressure created by the baby sucking. Having said this, some women experience none of these sensations yet have perfectly good let-down reflexes.

Making sure the let-down works properly and reliably

To make sure that your let-down works properly and reliably, check through the following points.

Be calm, unhurried, and enjoy the feeds

Have everything you need (for you, the baby and other children) to hand.

Decide in advance what you will do about the phone, the front door bell and other people who may be with you in the room (see page 118).

Cut out activities which worry you but are inessential, such as unnecessary entertaining, letter writing, telephoning, and cooking.

Cut down on other activities so that you always have time for feeds and are never in a hurry to do something else. This will mean that you don't promise to be anywhere at any set time but explain that you'll come when you're ready. Exceptions to this may have to be made, such as visits to your doctor.

Relax both before and during a feed by going through your relaxation technique learnt at ante-natal classes and by trying to clear your mind of any worries. While this sounds difficult, it'll come with practice.

Keep yourself fit

Make sure you are eating and drinking sensibly (see page 124).

Don't get overtired, and try to have at least one nap during the day if possible; put your feet up whenever you sit down; don't do unnecessary housework and other chores; organise shopping in the easiest way possible; and cut down on outside commitments for a while.

Condition your let-down reflex

Try to get into a routine before a feed – a regular chain of events will condition your let-down into working reliably.

Don't be tempted to skip night feeds: you need them to stimulate your milk supply.

When your breasts feel tense and full, wake the baby for a feed. Try not to let him sleep for long periods, because your breasts need regular emptying.

If your milk lets down unexpectedly, wake your baby and feed him.

Other points

Make sure you're comfortable when feeding – aching shoulders or a draught round your feet won't help.

If you have sore nipples, try to get your let-down to work before the baby feeds. Remember that the pain will eventually go and is anyway unlikely to last throughout a feed (see page 157).

A nasal spray containing synthetic oxytocin is available on prescription and will help your let-down if all else fails. Use this to give yourself confidence that you've got plenty of milk and then stop using it. Synthetic oxytocin constricts the small blood vessels in the lining of the nose and excessive use can damage the nasal lining causing ulceration.

Have a small alcoholic drink just before a feed. This will relax you and help your let-down (but see page 200).

Some mothers find a hot shower helps their let-down though this obviously isn't practical before every feed. Sometimes you might like to feed in the bath, where the warmth will encourage your milk to be let down.

There are several pitfalls to avoid when breastfeeding which you can't know about beforehand unless you've read a lot about breastfeeding and which may make you think your milk supply is poor.

One of the commonest reasons why women think they have insufficient milk is that they expect their babies to take exactly the same amount of milk at each feed. Should the baby want more than his mother can supply at one particular feed, she worries because she thinks she'll never be able to make enough milk for him again.

However, babies don't necessarily want the same amount to eat from feed to feed let alone from day to day. Your milk supply won't always necessarily match up with your baby's changing appetite, so be prepared that on some days he may be hungry. This happens to almost every mother and baby from time to time but is rarely mentioned in feeding manuals written for either mothers or professionals.

If your baby has previously been well satisfied with your milk but suddenly becomes edgy and miserable and you think he is still hungry after a feed, you must increase your milk supply to match his increased needs.

It's relatively easy for an inexperienced mother with an established breastfeeding pattern to panic if her baby seems to be unsatisfied by his feeds. Babies don't necessarily grow at a regular pace and may put on much more weight some weeks than others. Sometimes they'll grow so quickly that the mother's milk supply can't keep up with the increased demands, though this happens only if she tries to keep the feeds to the same number and length as they have been. The lesson is clear. If your milk supply has previously been adequate but your baby is now dissatisfied, let him suck for as long as he wants at each feed and give him as many feeds as he wants, as the odds are that he's having a *growth spurt* and your milk supply needs to be boosted by increasing the total time your baby spends at the breast. Growth spurts commonly occur at around six weeks and three months. If you're already feeding on demand, give him a couple of extra feeds during the day, or even more if you have time. The increased nipple stimulation will soon increase your milk production, though it will be several days before your supply catches up with his demand.

Another pitfall is that when you return home from hospital, whether it's at two or ten days, your milk supply is likely to dwindle temporarily because of the change, the excitement and the extra work you may find yourself doing. Family doctors say that they frequently receive calls from mothers just home saying that their milk has gone. Of course it hasn't gone for good and they can easily increase it; there's no need to give the baby a bottle or stop breastfeeding because of this temporary decrease in supply. If you realise the problem may crop up, you'll be able to cope better. Milk only dries up in a well-nourished woman if there is insufficient nipple stimulation and/or poor emptying of the breast. With enough of these, you can go on producing milk for years if you like. *The early drying up of milk is a man-made disorder, not a natural occurrence.*

Of course, the basic problem behind an inadequate milk supply *may be that your baby simply isn't milking your breast well enough for some reason.* Because of this, your nipples aren't stimulated adequately and you don't produce enough milk, even though you are quite capable of doing so and would have done from the beginning if your baby had milked you well from the start. All the time in the world spent with a baby who isn't performing optimally at the breast won't necessarily produce more milk but will tire you both out. When a baby milks optimally, your milk will be let down more efficiently and your breasts will be emptied more completely. There are many reasons why your baby may not be milking you well and correspondingly many ways of overcoming this problem (see page 187).

A well-tried technique for stimulating the milk supply by encouraging a baby to suck more strongly is switch nursing. All you do is switch the baby from one breast to the other several times during a feed, instead of just giving him each breast once per feed. A very young, tired, jaundiced, pethidine-doped, ill, pre-term or otherwise apathetic baby can often be coaxed into sucking better for longer this way.

Old wives' tales abound on the subject of increasing the milk supply and it's probably fair to say that when there are lots of conflicting old wives' tales, none is much good. There's no harm in following them, though, *provided you also carry out the* proven *methods above.* The danger comes when mothers rely solely on these fairytale methods of feeding successfully and forget the basic principles. Because you know someone for whom these old remedies worked, that doesn't mean that they'll work for you. By the time you've worked through even a small proportion of all the available 'cures', your milk will have gone for good.

Some tips you may be given are that vitamin B will work wonders – in fact its only probable benefit will be to make you feel well in yourself, though that may help indirectly; that alcohol, especially heavy beers, will help – again they may (in small amounts only), but only by making you relaxed and so aiding your let-down reflex; that vitamin E will increase your milk supply – there's no scientific proof of this; that drinking cows' milk will make more breast milk – quite wrong; that drinking more fluid than you actually need will make more milk – in fact it can do the opposite, the secret is to drink what you want; and that there are magic drugs which will increase your milk supply. Chlorpromazine, other phenothiazine drugs and the rauwolfia group of drugs do increase the milk supply but they should be used very much as a last resort, if at all. A new approach to stimulating the milk supply with drugs involves the use of metoclopramide, a drug normally used for gastric troubles and which was found to stimulate the secretion of prolactin. Small trials have shown that this does increase the milk supply but as with all drugs we have to ask ourselves what else it might be doing as well.

Adequacy of milk is not solely a concern of western women. Throughout the centuries women in many cultures have used amulets, potions, herbal skin rubs, chants and prayers to ensure they will have the right amount of milk. With our present knowledge of breastfeeding we know that these methods are unnecessary. By following the simple rules outlined above we can nearly always ensure that we will have enough milk for our babies without recourse to any magic. Indeed, moral support and reassurance are often all that are needed.

Cows' milk complements

If you were persuaded to let your baby have cows' milk complements as well as breast milk in hospital, don't worry. It's quite possible to start breastfeeding fully once you get home.

Reduce the amount of cows' milk formula by about half an ounce at each feed, so your baby will want more breast milk each time. Give the formula by spoon (or, if necessary, via a Lact-aid) rather than from a bottle.

We suggest using a spoon for complementary feeds because once your baby has become used to the different technique of drinking from a bottle, he'll be very loath to accept your nipple. Studies have shown that levels of breastfeeding can be raised by 50 per cent in hospitals allowing complementary feeds to be given only by spoon.

After two days of increased suckling time, letting the baby suck as much as he wants to even on an empty breast, your milk supply will begin to increase. Be prepared for at least two days of long and frequent feeds – perhaps as much as forty minutes every two hours or for longer periods with the baby sucking and napping on and off for several hours sometimes. Look after yourself by doing as few other things as possible – just rest and cuddle the baby. It's perfectly possible to build up your milk supply if you have the confidence and patience to do it (see also page 145).

What if all should fail?

If you've got this far in the book you'll have read enough to be thoroughly disappointed if you do 'fail' at breastfeeding. Unfortunately, with the best will in the world a very few women will be unable to breastfeed. Should you be one of these, don't despair – it's not the end of the world! After all, there is an alternative and such breastfeeding as you have been able to do will be better than nothing.

You may find that you'll have enough milk to give your baby the occasional feed – perhaps in the early morning. What's more, with the relief of your anxiety over starving him, your let-down might start working well and you may find you have more available milk than you thought.

The important thing is not to transfer your disappointment to your baby. It's certainly not his fault and it isn't yours either. Your attachment to and love for your child are more important than your milk.

If it comes to the crunch, a loving caring mother is what a baby really needs most so don't let things get so on top of you that you ruin your unique relationship. When you feed him with a bottle, hold him exactly as you did when breastfeeding and don't suddenly treat him like a doll, held at arm's length.

Increasing numbers of mothers who for some reason can't produce enough breast milk, either temporarily or permanently, are using a Lact-aid (see page 267) to enable their babies to feed at the breast and to get whatever milk there is at the same time as receiving cows' milk formula via a fine tube entering the baby's mouth along with the nipple. This gadget gives both mother and baby the pleasure of breastfeeding while assuring adequate nutrition.

If you ever have another baby, try again. You'll be a lot more confident as a mother and will have experience that is bound to help. Failure to breastfeed for as long as you wanted to the first time may mean that you need more help and back-up the next time. It's up to you to make sure you get it.

What if I don't want to carry on?

It's usually easy to make your milk dry up and it's not advisable to use dry-up pills. Simply reduce the length of time your baby spends at the breast by gradually cutting down the number amd length of feeds over a period of several weeks, if possible. Too rapid weaning may cause problems such as engorgement (see page 155) and blocked ducts and a breast infection can occur. As your baby gets less breast milk, give correspondingly more cows' milk formula by bottle or cup. Some mothers find that in order to produce enough milk to satisfy their babies they are having to spend more time with their babies at the breast than they are prepared to give up. Giving complementary bottles in this situation will ease the pressure for such mothers. Feeding a baby shouldn't be seen as a gruelling or annoying chore. If it is, then a mother is well advised to reconsider what she is doing.

It is better for the baby to have a happy mother who happens to be giving him cows' milk formula than an unhappy breastfeeding one who may get to the stage of being depressed or so uptight that physical battering becomes a possibility. Sometimes practical help can sustain a mother who finds her baby too time-consuming and tiring. It's wise not to be too proud to ask for such help if it might enable you to carry on breastfeeding.

Is the baby getting too much?

In the early days, before your milk supply has become established so that it matches your baby's demands, you may have too much milk for him. Over the days the supply will gradually adjust but the abundance can cause problems, especially towards the end of the first week. A newborn baby can be bewildered and almost choked by an over-exuberant flow of milk. He'll turn his head away, cough and splutter and be reluctant to go on feeding. He will also swallow too much air as he tries to drink from this 'fire hydrant' and this can produce colic. (See page 99).

You can cope with this by expressing some milk before a feed, either by hand or by letting the milk leak away if your let-down works before your baby is put to the breast.

If you allow your breasts to become overfull by letting your baby sleep too long between feeds, the same problem can arise. Wake him when your breasts feel full and tense, otherwise he'll be overwhelmed by the flow later.

Many women get over the problem of too much milk by feeding from one breast only at each feed (see page 175).

Your baby may prefer to feed in an 'uphill' position if your milk flows fast and furiously, as this may prevent the spray of milk from catching him in the back of his throat. Hold him facing you on your lap and then guide his head on to your breast, holding your nipple if necessary.

As your baby grows, he'll be better able to cope with an efficient, fast let-down reflex without choking. You should think yourself lucky if this is your 'problem' – better to have a good let-down than an unreliable, weak one.

If you have too much milk for your baby, think about donating the extra to a milk bank, where it would be used for premature or sick babies whose mothers didn't want to or couldn't breastfeed. Ask your doctor how to go about this in your area.

11 The working mother

When we talk to mothers about their reasons for *not* breastfeeding it isn't long before the subject of getting back to work crops up. Women have now become an important part of the work force in the western world and five million married women are employed in the UK. It's very difficult to find out exactly how many women with young children work because so many of them do part-time work or work at home and much of this is unrecorded by government agencies. In the USA in 1969 one in four women with children under three was working and in 1971 in the UK one in five women with children under four was working, though only one in twenty-five worked full-time.

We saw in Chapter 1 how young western women are brought up to think of themselves as important economic units and how this militates against breastfeeding. To many young women, their job comes first and raising children has to fit in with keeping up the family's standard of living. Having said this, such figures as are available show that only a tiny proportion of women are working when their children are of breastfeeding age.

Let's make no bones about it – full breastfeeding and work don't mix easily, if at all – at least not in this society. The International Labour Organisation has laid down rules to help mothers breastfeed in certain countries. It stipulates that nursing mothers should have a break of half an hour twice during the working day. These breaks are recognised in many countries and in some the breaks are shorter but more frequent. Two breaks during the day mean that a mother can feed before work, once during the morning, at lunch time, once during the afternoon and then at home in the evening and at night as much as necessary. In many countries employers must by law provide a room for breastfeeding mothers. In France, for instance, establishments employing more than 100 women over the age of fifteen must provide nurseries. In Denmark, if twenty-five or more women are employed, a breastfeeding room must be provided.

Breastfeeding at work is almost impossible for mothers in the UK as so few organisations have nurseries. In parts of Africa a baby is either brought to the working mother by relatives so that she can feed him or the mothers take their babies to work and actually have them by their sides as they work. Neither of these is likely to happen here!

But although it is difficult to combine breastfeeding and working, let's see how it can be done. First, though, we'll discuss why some women *want* to or have to combine the two.

Many mothers today say that living is so expensive that they simply can't afford to run a home on one income. That may seem to be the case but it's a thought that's worth challenging. Just think what you'd have to go without if you didn't work for nine months, for instance, and weigh up the advantages of being with your baby and feeding him yourself. Very often going back to work is shrouded in economic excuses when really the mother wants to keep in the swim and maintain her career or even simply her own original self-image – that is, the status quo. Mothers who take to mothering naturally don't want to leave their babies; they'll go through all sorts of hardships to stay at home. However, you don't necessarily realise what a pull your baby is going to be to make you want to stay at home until you've actually had it. Taking a part-time job to be 'released from the baby' or to 'keep up one's sanity' and all the other reasons mothers give is a sad but understandable reflection on today's society. With today's small family units and the inevitable isolation of mothers and babies at home, it's not really surprising that many mothers don't enjoy the experience of looking after their children and so try to find a way out.

In rural Africa a mother and her baby are not parted at all for the first fifteen months of life. A sample of these mothers was studied carefully to see if they became irritated by being with their children so closely for so long. No ill effects could be found in either the mothers or their babies. A popular myth is that babies need exposure to lots of different people to make them sociable. There's no evidence that this is so. Babies need their mothers and they need them most in the early years of life.

There is a small number of women for whom working is essential for the financial survival of the family and many more for whom the extra money would be helpful, so let's be practical and see how breastfeeding can be managed while working.

Obviously the easiest solution is to work at home doing something that makes money. There are all kinds of home-based jobs, from making things to telephone selling, which will enable you to carry on feeding naturally. The next best option is to work part-time and locally. Working locally not only cuts down on commuting time but also means that you can pop home in an emergency. If you work part-time you may like to express some breast milk to leave in the fridge for the baby minder to give your baby by bottle or by spoon while you are out.

Expressing milk (see page 94) is best done after each feed at home. Wash your hands well first. You'll probably only get a small volume of milk each time, but when it's all collected together there'll hopefully be enough for your baby while you're out. Some mothers manage to leave enough just by expressing their milk after the early morning feed, when the breasts are usually fuller than at any other time of the day. You'll soon learn what works best for you. Make sure that your minder knows how to shake and warm your baby's feed, and unless you're quite sure that you've left enough milk tell her what to give your baby if he's still hungry. Boiled, cooled water will fill his tummy until you get home. If he seems to need water, try to increase your milk supply so that you can leave more breast milk in future. Keep cows' milk formula complements as a very last resort.

Some mothers express milk while they're at work, store it in a fridge, take it home and it's ready for the baby minder to give to the baby the next day. The trouble with expressing is that it's rather tedious, usually takes longer than actually feeding the baby and needs privacy and somewhere comfortable to sit. When done in the morning it tends to be rushed because there's so much else to do, so either there may not be enough milk or else you may give up after a few days. If you are dedicated enough to carry on you'll have the satisfaction of knowing that your baby is fully breastfed.

Milk should be expressed into a previously sterilised plastic container, covered and then kept cold all the time (until being warmed for a feed). If you can't put your container of breast milk straight into a fridge at work, take a wide-necked Thermos flask with some ice in it to work and gently put your container into this.

Such a flask is also useful for taking your milk home.

If your breasts are uncomfortably full, express some milk and discard it if you don't want to take it home for your baby. If you let your breasts stay too full, you'll run the risk of getting a blocked duct, a breast infection, and of gradually losing your milk.

With local part-time work your baby will possibly need feeding only once while you're away. When you work some way away from home or when you're back full-time it requires effort and determination to leave enough expressed milk for the baby while you're away. You'll almost certainly have to express milk at work, keep it in a fridge there, and take it home for your baby to have the next day, as well as expressing milk after each feed at home. If you find that your milk supply is diminishing, remember that expressing milk by hand doesn't stimulate the breasts to produce as much milk as does the baby's sucking, so you may have to express more often or use a pump to make up for this.

If you decide you don't want to express milk at work, this doesn't mean you can't breastfeed at all. You can still feed before you go and as soon as you come back, besides at night. It's really tiring if you're getting up at night *and* working full-time, so bear this in mind when deciding to go back to work. Once you stop feeding on demand at home and expressing at work, your milk will probably slowly dry up, so with this sort of irregular feeding you'll gradually start weaning your baby whether you like it or not.

Many mothers who know that they're going to return to work worry about whether or not to get their baby used to a bottle before they go, to make things easier for the baby minder. It's probably best not to but to carry on with your normal breastfeeding behaviour right up until the day you go back to work. A hungry baby will take your expressed breast milk from a bottle if a minder gives it to him, but may quite understandably refuse it if you try to do it. Also, the later you can introduce the bottle, the better, as some babies soon learn to prefer the bottle to the breast (see page 172). Some babies will take expressed breast milk from a spoon.

When you're at home in the evenings, weekends or at other times on shift work, go back to feeding your baby on demand or even more often if you want to increase the milk supply or relieve the tension in your breasts. Frequent uncurtailed feeds at home, combined with relatively frequent expression of your milk at work, should keep your milk supply going effectively.

If you are a wage earner and a mother, you'll probably soon feel tired out, especially if you have other children as well as a breast-feeding baby. Babies often don't sleep in the early evenings, so you might like to carry him around in a sling to keep him happy while you're getting supper. Some working mothers encourage their babies to stay awake in the evenings so that they can spend some time with them.

Very few women actually give up breastfeeding to go back to work. In a study in Blackburn, only 0.6 per cent of women stopped for this reason. Those who really want to breastfeed carry on as long as they want and go back to work later at a time to suit themselves.

So, in summary, if you want to or have to work, do everything you possibly can to stay at home with your baby for at least three to six months, working at home if you can. After three to six months combine breast and bottle-feeding if you have to but carry on breastfeeding as long as you can, even if it's only one feed a day.

12 Some common problems

To say that each breastfeeding mother and each breastfed baby is different seems obvious. However, when it comes to a problem with breastfeeding, it's important to remember that each mother–baby pair needs individual advice. What works for one woman may work for another with a similar problem but sometimes women get round the same problem in different ways. If you can't work out what to do by yourself, get some help from a counsellor experienced in helping large numbers of mothers and babies. Not only does the age and the birth history of the baby influence the situation, but also the personalities of the mother and the baby, the home environment, other advice being given at the same time, and the expectations of the mother and father.

Engorgement (swollen, tender breasts)

As your colostrum alters to become mature milk in the first few days it's very important that your breasts are emptied frequently (though not necessarily completely) enough to prevent them becoming overfilled.

If you don't put your baby to your breasts enough, milk will build up until they become swollen, lumpy, hard, tense, painful and hot. This is called engorgement and is due not only to the excess milk but also to the swelling caused by the increased blood supply and by leakage of fluid from lymphatic and blood vessels blocked by the increased pressure in the breasts. This fluid collects under the skin and in the connective tissues. The skin of engorged breasts is liable to bruise and is shiny and pitted like orange peel.

Added to this, the swollen ducts and milk reservoirs can often be seen standing out as lumps and 'cords' beneath the skin.

A mother with engorgement feels hot and shivery and may sweat profusely. She often feels thirsty and should drink according to her thirst, and not limit drinks as she may be advised to do. Some mothers feel weepy when they have engorged breasts. This may be because of the discomfort or may be because engorgement often coincides with the low period often noticed towards the end of the first week, Some experts go so far as to say that if mothers didn't get engorged breasts they wouldn't become depressed post-natally.

But discomfort is only a part of the problem. The milk-producing cells within the milk glands are also affected by the high pressure in the breasts. They become flattened and unable to produce so much milk. While this may be a good thing in the short term, in that it reduces milk production and so reduces further build-up of pressure in the breasts, it's a very bad thing in the long term, because the ability of the cells to produce milk can be damaged so much that milk production is shut down altogether. (NB. This is not to say that they can *never* produce milk again).

This is the method most hospitals use to dry up milk in mothers who don't want to feed their babies. They are advised not to feed and their milk simply goes. They become engorged toward the end of the first week, as their milk comes in even without their babies feeding at the breast but, because of the build-up of pressure in their breasts, the milk-producing cells are so damaged that they stop producing milk at all. With no further stimulus from suckling and thus no hormone release, the milk dries up.

The breastfeeding mother with a good let-down reflex is lucky as, if she does become engorged, by breastfeeding properly she can restore the milk-producing cells to their former healthy state, so that when she has managed to get rid of the engorgement her milk production will be as good as before. If she were to carry on breastfeeding halfheartedly, the engorgement might be relieved but her milk production might never again regain its former potential and would eventually dry up.

Poor management of engorgement is one of the commonest reasons for failure of the milk supply in the early days, yet this failure should be entirely preventable. Mothers who say that their milk vanished after a week could in almost every case have breastfed successfully if only they had been given better advice.

If you follow the advice earlier in the book about how to manage breastfeeding in the first few days, *it's unlikely that you will become engorged at all.* However, if you have been given poor advice (and one leading American doctor says that in his opinion engorgement is a disorder caused by doctors!) then this is how to cope with the engorgement and lay the foundations for successful breastfeeding in the months ahead:

1 Feed your baby more often and feed him as soon as your breasts feel at all full, even if he hasn't asked for a feed and is asleep.

2 Feed your baby for longer periods.

3 If your breasts are so tense that it's difficult for your baby to feed, soften the areola beforehand by removing some milk. You can do this in one of several ways: by gently expressing a little milk by hand (if this is not too painful); by having a hot bath to encourage leaking; by splashing your breasts with warm water over a hand basin; by using a breast pump; or by encouraging your let-down to work by relaxing, going through the routine of preparing to feed or by taking an aspirin or a small alcoholic drink to reduce any pain which may be stopping you from letting down your milk. A baby that is allowed to suck on a tense areola will be unlikely to get the breast into his mouth properly, will chew on a small part of the nipple and will not only make the nipple sore but also get very little milk. This is because he is not able to drain the milk reservoirs, and the pain he is causing by chewing on the nipples prevents the let-down from working.

4 If your baby is too apathetic (see page 170) to empty the breasts enough to get rid of the painful lumpiness when he has finished feeding, you can empty them either by hand expression or with an electric or hand breast pump. There is no need to empty them fully.

The widely available hand pump with a rubber bulb and a glass container is not very effective or comfortable. Suitable hand pumps which you can buy are listed in the Appendix. Electric pumps are preferred by some mothers to hand expression. These are very expensive to buy but can be rented from a variety of sources, including some National Childbirth Trust branches and La Leche League groups, hospitals and medical supply houses. The various pumps available differ slightly in their action. The Egnell pump closely imitates the baby's sucking action, while the Whittlestone pump 'milks' the breast and can pump from both breasts at once, so halving the time taken. Care must be taken when using any pump to follow the instructions for cleaning and use. Your milk may flow better if you start the let-down by expressing some milk first, and if you change from side to side every so often (as you do when hand expressing or encouraging a baby to keep sucking). As long as your nipples don't become sore, gradually increase the length of time you spend pumping.

5 The tenderness and pain of engorged breasts can be relieved with ice packs, with hot or cold compresses (made by wringing out a flannel in hot or cold water) applied as often as necessary, or by splashing with warm or cold water.

Sore and painful nipples

Many breastfeeding mothers experience pain in their nipples during the early weeks of breastfeeding, particularly in the first week, and unfortunately this pain puts many of them off completely. Various surveys have estimated that between 13 and 80 per cent of mothers have sore nipples at some time.

Although it's not always possible to prevent the nipples becoming painful, it is possible to prevent the condition from lasting too long or from getting worse.

What causes the pain? There is some dispute about this, especially as in some women the nipple skin itself is undamaged. In others, the nipple skin is visibly roughened, usually with reddening and raising of the small projections (papillae) of the nipples together with a crescentic stripe of 'petechiae' – tiny spots of blood within the skin – across each nipple. Crusting of the skin can also occur.

The pain from a sore nipple begins as soon as the baby starts feeding and generally lasts only a minute or two, not throughout the feed. In mothers feeding their babies on demand, the peak of nipple soreness occurs on the third day and by the fourth day it is decreasing, whereas in mothers feeding their babies on a four-hourly schedule, the soreness continues to get worse until the fourth day. Babies fed on a schedule may damage the nipple skin more as they suck more strongly because they are so hungry. Large babies tend to cause more soreness than small ones, for the same reason.

The pain is very characteristic and is described as being as though the baby were biting the nipple. It usually goes as soon as the milk is let down and it is perhaps for this reason that it is always less or even non-existent in the 'second' breast.

The most reasonable explanation for the pain, with or without actual skin damage, would seem to be the strong suction exerted on the nipple by the baby's mouth before the milk is let down. Very high negative pressures are produced in his mouth during this time and these are the cause of the skin damage described above. The crescentic stripe represents the area of the nipple exposed to maximum suction, the baby's palate resting above the stripe and his tongue below. Mothers who have no visible skin damage may have tougher nipple skin which is more resistant to the suction exerted. The pain stops (provided that the nipple skin is not too damaged) when the let-down reflex operates because the supply of milk means the baby no longer needs to suck so strongly.

When the milk is being produced freely, towards the end of the first week after birth, there is always some foremilk available for the baby when he is put to the breast and extreme pressure causing damage to the skin from sucking empty milk reservoirs should not occur.

In the occasional mother who experiences soreness of the nipples in later weeks, it is possible that the foremilk is not getting to the baby as soon as he sucks. This may be because her ducts are kept closed because she is cold, in which case she should either have a warm shower or bath before feeding or bathe her breasts with warm water. She should also feed in a warm room and wear warm clothes.

A baby who has the nipple and areola positioned poorly in his mouth, because of being held awkwardly or because his mother has poorly protractile nipples or engorgement of the breast, is more likely to cause soreness due to skin damage.

Nipple soreness can be extremely painful as any experienced breastfeeding mother knows. Don't be surprised if you wince at the beginning of a feed or even cry out: this doesn't mean that you have a low pain threshold or that you're a coward. Just remember that nipple soreness can be cured. As the days go by, the skin on your nipples will anyway grow tougher and more pain-resistant. When you stop breastfeeding, you'll notice that your nipple skin will return to its former state.

What can be done to treat sore nipples?

The cardinal rule is to carry on feeding: *don't stop*, whatever you're told.

1 *First of all and very important, make sure that your baby is positioned well at the breast.* If your nipple skin looks sore, with a stripe across it, it's highly likely that he is feeding with his mouth in an awkward position, so exerting unnecessary suction on the nipple to hold it in place. Sit up or even lean slightly forward, making sure that the baby is not tugging at the nipple but is well supported. Put the baby's chest against yours so he doesn't have to turn his head to get to the breast and make sure his chin is against your breast. He should have part or all of the areola (depending on its size) in his mouth, and certainly not just the nipple itself. Change the position in which you feed your baby during the day. A good tip is to feed him in the 'normal' position on your lap and with you sitting up for all the morning feeds after you've got up; with him in the 'football hold' position (his legs pointing under the arm of the side you're feeding him from and his body supported by a cushion if necessary) and you sitting up during the afternoon and evening; and with him lying down at your side during the night. With a little thought you can work out other variations of position. Some mothers learn the knack of lying by their baby at night and feeding him from the breast opposite to the side he's lying on by leaning over him carefully and half lying on their tummy.

Changing your feeding position regularly ensures that no single part of the nipple takes the force of his suction every time.

2 *If your nipples are poorly protractile* try using breast shells for half an hour or so before a feed. These may make the nipples temporarily stand out enough for the baby to take them better. Be careful to keep the shells clean to avoid introducing infection into the damaged skin. A word of warning here. Breast shells can make the nipple skin swollen and moist because of the still, warm, air inside them. This may itself cause more soreness and can also make a crack of the nipple skin worse. Whether or not the shells help is an individual matter and the thing is to try them once or twice to see if they help you.

3 *If you are engorged,* treat this as described on page 154 A baby will

find it difficult to feed in the correct position from an engorged breast and is very likely to chew the nipple as the areola may be too tense to be taken into his mouth.

4 Fear of pain, as well as actual pain, delays the let-down reflex, which means that the baby will carry on sucking strongly and your nipples will be painful for longer. Try to *encourage* your let-down to work before the baby is put to the breast by going through a set routine of preparing for a feed.

5 *Feed your baby frequently.* This will encourage the milk to come in sooner and will also aid the establishment of your let-down reflex. You may develop sore nipples sooner than your schedule-feeding neighbour in the next bed but the soreness will also disappear before hers, your breastfeeding will almost certainly be more successful and you will be less likely to develop mastitis from a blocked duct and/or infection.

6 *Don't limit drinking time but limit total suckling time.* Suckling to comfort your baby while he goes to sleep after he's finished drinking is good practice when your nipples are *not* sore but you may find it helps healing if you take him off the breast at this stage if you have sore nipples. By doing this and by encouraging your let-down to work before he feeds (number 4 above) you'll limit his total sucking time but not his actual drinking time. When your nipple soreness has eased after a day or two, go back to letting your baby suck for as long as he wants, or your milk supply may start diminishing.

7 *Care for your nipple skin* as described on page 96 and be careful not to soak your nipples in the bath water for too long. Moisture makes soreness last longer, especially if the baby feeds on soggy nipple skin, as the skin is more liable to damage after being soaked.

8 Some authorities recommend using antiseptic cream on sore nipple skin to help prevent a fissure developing. However, any cream will tend to trap water or leaking milk on the nipples, and sore nipples should be kept dry. Reserve antiseptic cream for if you get an *infected* nipple crack.

In the UK many women use an antiseptic (chlorhexidine) aerosol spray on their nipples in the mistaken belief that it will prevent nipple soreness, nipple cracks and mastitis. There is no evidence, however, to suggest that this spray prevents soreness or cracks or that it is effective against them once they have developed. Provided sensible breastfeeding techniques are used and that adequate precautions are taken against cross-infection in hospital, there is absolutely no reason to use such a spray.

9 *Always offer the less sore nipple first.* By the time you offer the sore one, your milk should be flowing well and there should be little pain.

10 To help you during the first part of a feed when your nipples feel most sore, try some breathing exercises and other relaxation techniques such as you learnt to help you cope with your labour.

11 *Take an aspirin or a small alcoholic drink* a short time before a feed if you feel the pain is inhibiting your let-down.

12 Careful use of ultra-violet light from a *sun lamp* (or an ultra-violet bulb in any lamp socket) can speed up the healing of damaged nipple skin. You should be three or four feet away from the lamp and your eyes should be protected by goggles or a thick towel. Expose your nipples for half a minute on the first day, one minute on days two and three, two minutes on days four and five and three minutes on day six. If there is any reddening of the skin, reduce the exposure time. If you can sunbathe with your nipples exposed, the sunlight will help a lot, but don't get sunburnt! If you have no garden, sunbathe indoors with the window open. Failing a sun lamp or sunlight, try exposing your nipple to the light from a sixty watt electric light bulb for twenty minutes two or three times a day.

13 *Don't remove any crusts* appearing on the nipples – they are part of the healing process.

14 Some people advocate using a rubber *nipple shield* over the sore nipple. This has a teat for the baby to suck your milk through. It may or may not help – try it only if all the other measures fail. One danger is that if not properly cleaned between times it can introduce infection into the damaged skin. It's important not to use a shield for long because milk production and the establishment of the let-down depend on actual skin stimulation by the baby (see also page 171).

15 It may help if you cool your nipples immediately before you put your baby to the breast. Try putting some *ice cubes* into a small polythene bag or a flannel and holding it against your nipple.

16 A very successful and simple hint for helping damaged nipple skin to heal is to express some milk after each feed, rub it on to the nipples and let it dry.

17 If you have to stop your baby from feeding, break the suction by putting the tip of a finger in the corner of his mouth. Just pulling him off may increase any soreness.

18 Last, but by no means least, is to *expose your nipples to the air* as much as possible. You may think this is difficult in a cold climate and in our culture, but you can sleep naked at night and leave your bra off during the day to allow the air to circulate under your top clothes. Once the soreness has healed, wear your bra again.

Air helps tremendously because it dries the nipple skin. If sore nipple skin is allowed to remain moist after a feed, the soreness will persist. Moisture also makes cracking and infection more likely. When you wear a bra again, dry your nipples before covering them, and if you use anything inside your bra to mop up leaks, make sure it is changed frequently to stop the nipples being enclosed in soggy material for long periods.

Some women have successfully used a piece of one-way nappy liner or absorbent paper inside their bra cups. This helps keep the nipples dry. Waterproof-backed bra pads are not ideal as they retain moisture next to the skin and encourage nipple soreness.

Rarely, a sore nipple may bleed and the baby may swallow tiny amounts of blood. This can look horrifying if it's regurgitated in a mouthful of milk but there's no need to worry. Your blood is quite harmless to the baby. Treat the soreness and carry on feeding.

If nipple soreness persists for the whole feed, consider whether it may be caused by dermatitis from detergents used to wash clothing or from substances in creams or other remedies applied to your nipples. Once the cause has been tracked down, remove it and treat the nipples with hydrocortisone cream from your doctor if necessary.

Thrush (an infection with the fungus or yeast *Candida albicans* –

also known as monilia) can infect the skin of the nipple and areola and cause soreness. The source of thrush is usually the mouth of the newborn baby. The baby is likely to have caught it during his passage down the birth canal because thrush is a relatively common infection of the vagina and vulva in pregnant (and breastfeeding) women. The fungus thrives in warm, moist situations and seems to like milk, so the baby's mouth and the mother's nipple and areola area (particularly if encased in a bra pad and bra) make very suitable breeding grounds. It's very easy for the mother and baby to pass thrush backwards and forwards to each other and it's important to make sure that both are treated simultaneously, promptly and vigorously. If the mother has vaginal thrush (monilial vulvo-vaginitis), that should be treated at the same time as well. A home remedy for thrush in the baby's mouth is sodium bicarbonate solution, made by dissolving a level teaspoon of sodium bicarbonate in a cup of water. Swab the inside of your baby's mouth thoroughly after each feed with this solution, using a cotton wool ball. Make a new solution each day and use a clean swab each time. At the same time, thrush on your nipples can be treated after each feed with a vinegar solution made by mixing a teaspoon of vinegar with one cup of water. Sunshine or ultra-violet light from a sunlamp or an ultra-violet bulb (used with strict precautions, see page 161) may help get rid of thrush on your nipples as well.

There is no need to stop breastfeeding. If it is necessary to get help from your doctor, he may prescribe nystatin. The baby's mouth should be carefully rinsed with water after each time at the breast and a little (1 ml) of the nystatin suspension dripped by a dropper into his mouth. The mother should wash her nipples and areolae after each feed, dry them well, then put some nystatin ointment on to the skin. New bra pads must be worn then.

The baby can become reinfected from anything that has previously been in his mouth, so take care to boil daily for twenty minutes any dummy or rubber teat you may have given him. Thrush in the baby's mouth looks like patches of milk curds but, unlike milk curds, cannot be scraped off the mouth lining without making it bleed. Treatment of both mother and baby is best carried out for two weeks even if both seem better beforehand.

Nipple cracks (fissures)

A few women develop a fissure or crack in the nipple usually after the fifth day. This develops at the base of the nipple and may follow poor treatment of the more usual nipple soreness described above. A crack usually develops in the line across the nipple where the baby applies maximum suction while feeding. Prevent it reopening by regularly changing your baby's feeding position (see page 159). A fissure is acutely painful and needs careful and prompt treatment if the pain is not going to put you off breastfeeding altogether. Thrush, possibly from the baby's mouth, may infect a fissure and needs special treatment (see above).

The best prevention and treatment for a fissure is to take all the steps for the treatment of sore nipples. Letting some expressed milk dry on your nipples after each feed speeds up healing markedly. If, however, you have a fissure which doesn't heal with this treatment within a few days, you'll probably find it necessary to take the baby off the breast because of the pain and either express the milk or use an electric pump for a while – sometimes as long as four or five days, though usually for only one or two. Give your milk to the baby by spoon. Avoid using a bottle as some babies find it difficult to suck at the breast afterwards. When the fissure has healed, gradually resume feeding your baby, starting twice a day and continuing to pump or express regularly in between feeds. Some mothers find they can continue to feed if they use a rubber nipple shield but, again, great care must be taken to keep it clean and to stop using it as soon as possible.

Blocked duct (causing a swollen, tender area)

This causes a red, tender lump or area in the breast. The duct becomes blocked either because of pressure from part of a badly fitting bra or from generalised engorgement of the breast with inadequate emptying of one duct in particular. Milk builds up in the duct behind the blockage and causes a lump. When the baby feeds, the let-down works even in the area of the breast supplying the blocked duct, so the pressure builds up more, often making the lump most painful as the milk lets down. If a blocked duct is treated at this stage, the lumpy area will subside with no further problem. If nothing is done, the affected part of the breast becomes inflamed because milk escapes from the duct into the surrounding tissues of the breast and also causes reddening of the overlying skin. Inflammatory products get into the bloodstream and make the body temperature rise. This can cause a fever as high as $104°F$ ($40°C$) after a feed! The mother may feel flu-like and achey as well. Inflammation of part or all of the breast, with or without infection, is known as mastitis.

Treatment of a blocked duct should be regarded as urgent because stagnant milk in the gland and duct behind the blocked duct, and in the surrounding breast tissue, can so easily become infected. Simple measures, started at the first suspicion that anything is wrong, should do the trick in every case.

1 Make sure the whole breast is emptied thoroughly each time your baby feeds. Complete emptying is normally unnecessary but, in the case of the blocked duct, the lower the tension of milk in the breast, the more chance you have of clearing the blockage. Let your baby feed as long as he wants and then express any residual milk.

2 Should your breasts or even a part of a breast still feel lumpy after a feed, feed the baby more often to ensure frequent drainage of the ducts. Try to fit in as many extra feeds as you can, even if you are already feeding on demand.

3 Offer the affected breast first to ensure the best possible emptying and return to it later on in the feed.

4 *Gently* but firmly massage the lump towards the nipple during a feed (and after if it is still there) in an attempt to release the milk.

5 Check that your bra is not pressing anywhere and so causing the block, especially if you're using one of the nursing bras that has a band across the top of the breast when the flap is open, or if you are pulling the cup of an ordinary bra down to feed.

6 Vary the position of your baby at each feed (see page 159). This simple tip is one of the most helpful.

7 Relieve the pain with hot wet compresses applied every hour or put a hot water bottle over the area. Splashing the breast with hot

water while leaning over a basin before a feed may help or, even better, immerse your breasts in comfortably hot water for five to ten minutes.

8 If the lump is still present after twenty-four hours in spite of all these measures, it's wise to take a course of antibiotics to prevent infection, so go and see your doctor. *You shouldn't stop feeding*.

9 Make sure you get plenty of rest. Actually go to bed; even if it's only for one day it will make you feel better and may help keep your resistance up so that your blocked duct won't lead to mastitis.

10 If you are a fairly inactive person, physical exercise, especially of the shoulders, arms and upper half of the body, may help disperse a painful swelling caused by a blocked duct.

Some women have noticed that if they try to express milk from a blocked duct, they can eventually produce a small firm 'plug' of white or yellow, cheesy or granular matter from the opening of that duct at the nipple. This plug is probably made of the milk that has been dammed up for longest behind the blockage from outside the duct. The milk that is then expressed from that duct is usually thick and may flow slowly of its own accord for a while. When this milk that was in the blocked duct and gland has all been expressed, the newly produced milk looks quite normal. The thickening of the milk is simply due to stasis and water absorption. Such women are liable to have repeated blockages which may respond to a dietary change. One American obstetrician suggests that polyunsaturated fats should be substituted for saturated fats, and extra lecithin included in the diet.

Breast infection (mastitis with infection)

Poor or delayed treatment of a blocked duct can lead to infection of the inflamed breast. The infection usually starts in milk which has escaped from the duct into the surrounding breast tissue due to pressure within the duct as more milk is let down. Sometimes pus can be expressed from the duct at the nipple.

The appearance of an infected breast differs only in degree from that of the breast with a blocked duct. The infected area is red, swollen, hot and painful, with shiny skin, and the mother feels shivery and flu-like as before. She may also feel nauseated.

The treatment of this sort of breast infection is as for a blocked duct, with the addition of an antibiotic. There is *no* danger to the baby from drinking the milk, as the organisms responsible are not harmful and in any case are rarely present in the milk.

Don't be tempted or persuaded to wean your baby – if you do you'll be likely to develop a breast abscess.

This sort of mastitis, known as *sporadic mastitis*, is most often seen after several weeks of breastfeeding. Occasionally it occurs without a duct being blocked, apparently out of the blue.

Epidemic mastitis is another type of infection which is passed to the breast from the baby via the nipple and causes illness in the first two weeks or so of feeding. The organisms responsible often come from the hospital nursery and are carried in the baby's nose. Several mothers and babies may be affected at once in a hospital, hence the name 'epidemic' mastitis.

The infection involves the milk ducts (not the tissues outside the ducts as with infection following a blocked duct) and it is often possible to squeeze pus from the nipple. The *whole* breast is red, hot, tender and swollen and the mother feels feverish and ill.

The organisms responsible are from a more virulent strain of *Staphylococcus aureus* than that causing sporadic mastitis and may be sensitive to one of the newer penicillins, though some are penicillin-resistant. A milk sample should be cultured by the laboratory to determine which antibiotic is most suitable. The baby will probably come to no harm from drinking the infected milk if you are taking antibiotics, but some researchers suggest that milk with large numbers of dead or alive bacteria may produce a toxic or irritant effect (such as gastroenteritis or even septicaemia) in the baby and that the milk should not be drunk, even after being sterilised. A mother's milk, even if infected with these organisms, is probably tolerated better by her own baby than by someone else's. To be absolutely safe in cases of epidemic mastitis, a sample of milk should be examined and if found to contain a high bacteria count the baby should only be fed from the other breast or should have milk from another mother, or cows' milk formula if no breast milk is available. The breast should be emptied well and often by expression or pumping to maintain the milk supply and you should rest as much as possible. Treat the pain with aspirin and hot compresses and relax as much as you can before a feed to aid your let-down. If the bacteria count of the milk is within safe limits, or when it drops to safe limits, breastfeeding can be continued, but until then the milk should be discarded.

Breast abscess

This is usually preventable as it follows mastitis which has been poorly treated. One survey showed that *abscesses occurred only in women who stopped feeding when they got mastitis*. The lump is not tender.

Treatment is as for epidemic mastitis but if the abscess doesn't resolve, surgical drainage will be necessary. You can feed the baby from the affected breast if you and your doctor are reasonably sure that the infection is contained within the abscess (which is usually the case). Otherwise, carry on feeding with the other breast and temporarily discard the expressed milk from the one with the abscess.

After this catalogue of horrors the reader could be forgiven for thinking that she's going to have all kinds of unpleasant problems with swollen breasts and abscesses. This of course is unlikely.

The complications we've mentioned here are uncommon (except for sore nipples) and almost unknown in women who breastfeed in a natural way right from the beginning. A doctor we know who worked in a totally breastfeeding hospital unit in Africa saw no mastitis or breast abscesses in four years of looking after several thousand mothers.

Contrast this with the western world where an average of 9 per cent of breastfeeding mothers get mastitis, 5 to 11 per cent of whom suffer from breast abscesses.

Lump in the breast

Women of all ages and at all stages of their reproductive lives can get a lump in the breast. The important thing to remember is that breastfeeding is no sure protection against getting lumps so if you are in the habit of feeling your breasts for lumps each month (which is highly advisable) go on doing so while you are feeding. It will be more difficult to feel lumps if your breasts are larger and firmer, but if you feel one do take it seriously. Having said this, the lactating breast is often lumpy but the lumps are 'here today and gone tomorrow'. A significant breast lump will be there for days.

The causes of lumps during breastfeeding are much as at any other time but causes related to the production of milk come highest on the list, not surprisingly. A blocked duct causes a lump which should disappear in a few days with suitable treatment (see page 164). Lumps that are commonly found in the breast may well appear for the first time during lactation and need medical attention. In the majority of cases (four out of five) such lumps are not cancers and can be removed (preferably under local anaesthetic) and breastfeeding continued. A woman who develops a true cancer while feeding will probably be advised to wean because the therapy required to give her the best possible outcome is unlikely to be compatible with continuing breastfeeding.

A galactocele (milk retention cyst) is a non-tender, smooth, rounded, cystic swelling filled with milk that is thought to be caused in the first place by a blocked duct. If the cyst had become infected, it would have formed an abscess. If a blocked duct is treated with antibiotics but a faulty breastfeeding technique is continued, a sterile cyst can result. Sometimes gentle expression can empty the milk via the nipple. If nothing is done, the milk in the cyst gradually becomes thicker and creamy, cheesy or oily. If the cyst is aspirated, it will fill with milk again. It can be surgically removed under a local anaesthetic. Breastfeeding can be continued quite safely.

Difficult feeders

Some babies take to the breast within a few minutes of being born and never give their mothers any trouble. Others, however, seem completely uninterested, feed briefly, then let go and cry, or even seem to have a battle with the breast. In nearly every case there is a reason for the baby's behaviour. Whatever the cause of the difficulty with feeding, make sure that you keep your milk supply going. Though a few babies never feed enthusiastically, they all feed eventually if given the chance. The feeding of an unenthusiastic baby may not be enough to stimulate your milk supply, so it's up to you to express or pump after each feed. You may need to keep this up for some weeks, so be prepared. Let's look at the most common possible causes in turn.

Babies affected by mother's pain-killers in labour
In the UK pethidine is a common offender, while in the USA many babies are affected by barbiturates given to the mother in labour. These babies may be drowsy and apathetic about feeding for up to five days, though the effects usually wear off more quickly. Good obstetric care includes not giving large doses of pain-killers shortly before the birth. Some obstetric units hardly ever use pain-killers during labour but rely instead on breathing and other relaxation techniques, adequate support from a sympathetic and skilled birth attendant and, most important, on encouraging the mother to adopt an upright position (or whatever other position is best for her) in the first and second stages.

You might not be able to get your sedated baby to feed well but you can stop him being given a bottle and you can keep your milk supply going by expressing or pumping your breasts after each feed. You can also try giving him expressed milk from a spoon when he has finished feeding. Wake him often – every two or three hours at least – for a feed, as the sooner he learns how to feed from your breast, the better. While you or a nurse may be able to get him to suck from a bottle even if he won't feed from you, this isn't a good idea as he'll be far less likely to take to the breast once the sedation has worn off.

The keynote to managing this problem is perseverance but you can cope if you know what to do.

Poor feeding position
If the baby is not correctly positioned at the breast, the nipple will not be taken far enough into the mouth and the stimulus to feed will not be strong enough. See page 91 to make sure you are giving him the best chance to feed properly.

Poorly protractile nipples
A few mothers still have poorly protractile nipples at the end of their pregnancies, though these tend to improve once the baby has been suckled for several weeks. You'll find it helps to wear breast shells

for half an hour or so before a feed; this brings the nipples out just long enough for the baby to get a hold. A similar effect can be produced by a breast pump. Once he has 'latched on', the nipple should stay out for the length of the feed. When he stops feeding, it'll go back in.

You can also help your baby to latch on by taking your nipple and areola between your finger and thumb and making a 'biscuit' for him to take hold of. The 'biscuit' should be held so that it is parallel with the line of the baby's lips and not at right angles to it.

A rubber nipple shield can help in some cases in the early days but should be discarded as soon as possible as the nipples need the stimulus of sucking (see page 161).

Engorgement
(See page 154.)

Tired baby
If you are made to feed your baby according to a schedule in hospital, he may cry from hunger for some time – perhaps as long as an hour – before you are given him to feed. This is especially likely to happen at visiting times and at night. By the time you get him he is exhausted and goes to sleep after feeding for a very short time, even sometimes before your milk lets down.

Obviously this situation is ridiculous. You must insist that you are given your baby as soon as he cries. Remember that the smaller the baby, the more often he'll need feeding and the sooner crying will exhaust him.

Full baby
If your baby is given a cows' milk complement after you have fed him, he is unlikely to be hungry by the time the hospital decrees he's ready for a feed from you. This is because cows' milk formula stays in the stomach for much longer than breast milk. You'll know by this stage that complements are rarely, if ever, necessary in the first weeks, so tell the nurse that you would rather feed your baby more often and for longer and that you don't want him to have anything other than breast milk to drink, day or night. Remember that you need your baby to feed often so that your milk comes in quickly and

so that you produce enough milk for him. A baby full of cows' milk formula is no help to your breasts as he simply won't feed.

Baby kept from you after birth

The best time to start suckling is in the first half an hour after birth. After this the baby's urge to feed gradually lessens, though of course you can still teach him with patience. Learning to feed is best done in the first few hours; after that you'll have a much slower pupil on your hands.

Jaundiced baby (see also page 181)

A jaundiced baby is often sleepy and difficult to interest in feeding. Frequent small feeds are the best for him. As the jaundice clears, his interest will increase, so be patient and maintain your milk supply by expressing after each feed if necessary (see page 75).

Baby has been given a bottle

A baby who has sucked from a rubber teat will find it more difficult to feed from you as the rubber teat is a 'supernormal' stimulus. A baby who has learnt to bottle-suck will try to breastfeed using the same technique. Unfortunately it just doesn't work at the breast and the baby will have to relearn how to milk the breast. You can get him to feed from you with patience but try to keep him away from the bottle completely in the first place. Once a baby has fed from the breast for many weeks, the occasional experience of sucking from a rubber teat shouldn't matter, though some babies very quickly learn that milk comes from a bottle more easily and are reluctant to take the breast if there's the slightest chance of getting a bottle.

The technique a baby uses for bottle-sucking is very much easier than that which he uses when sucking at the breast. When being bottle-fed, the baby applies a little suction, lets the milk pour into his mouth and swallows it. There is little up and down or in and out movement of his tongue and less jaw movement. When a baby breastfeeds, the nipple and part of the areola are sucked in to his mouth, the front of his tongue is stuck out beneath the nipple as far as his lower lip and curled up slightly, then the back of the tongue is pushed up against the nipple and areola. The whole tongue moves back into the baby's mouth, pressing against the nipple and areola as it does so, and milking the milk out of the reservoirs beneath the areola. The baby's jaws open and close during this milking action to help the tongue compress the nipple and areola. The actual sucking involved is relatively unimportant though the suction by the cheeks is measurable. If a baby bottle-sucks the breast, he gets very little milk. There is much more effort involved in feeding from the breast and it's not surprising that the muscular effort expended is good for the development of the baby's jaws. If you are trying to teach a baby to breastfeed once he's been given a bottle, it's no help to him at all if you constantly muddle him by giving both the breast *and* bottle. If you want to breastfeed, don't give your baby a bottle at all. If for some reason he isn't getting all his nourishment direct from the breast, give him complements of expressed breast milk (or cows' milk formula) by spoon or from a Lact-aid (see page 208). Babies who know only how to bottle-suck can be spotted at the breast by the occasional indrawing of their cheeks caused by sucking their tongue, by their 'tongue thrusting' and by their ineffective (sometimes fluttering) sucking action. Feeds are long drawn out because their poor milking action doesn't encourage the let-down of the milk. Intervals between bouts of sucking are longer than usual and they don't swallow very often. Even one bottle can make subsequent feeding behaviour difficult. In the rare event of a mother being so ill that she can't feed her baby, the baby should be given his milk from a spoon (or from another mother), but *not* by bottle.

Baby fights at the breast

A baby who fights at the breast may have had the experience of being smothered by the full breast while feeding and has learnt that, for him, getting milk means not getting air through his nose. Make sure that your breast is not obstructing his nose. You may have to hold your breast away with your opposite hand holding the areola with two fingers like a cigarette. With patience on your part he'll forget his early unpleasant experience.

Don't confuse fighting at the breast with the common fussing or playing and butting some babies do while they're waiting for the milk to let down. These babies are perfectly happy once the milk is flowing, whereas the true fighters carry on fighting and never seem to feed properly.

If your baby is still reluctant to take the breast, try the trick of popping a rubber teat, perhaps filled with expressed milk, into his mouth. Once he latches on, withdraw it and substitute your nipple.

Baby refuses one breast

Occasionally a baby will seem to take a liking to one breast and refuse to feed from the other. This may be because he is more comfortable on one side or because the milk seems to come more easily from that breast. To overcome this, try feeding him from the side he likes best first, so that the milk is flowing from the other side, then transfer him to the other breast without turning him round, so letting him feed in the 'twin' position. This may do the trick. If not, express milk from the unused breast to maintain its milk supply and keep trying at each feed time. He'll also certainly come round to the idea of feeding from both sides again. Many babies (and, come to that, many mothers) prefer one side to the other. It's quite possible to end up rather lopsided if you feed your baby more at one side than the other. The side which isn't stimulated as much will respond by producing less milk in time. Some women have breasts which are unequal in size before they become pregnant. This doesn't matter at all, though they may find that they always seem to have more milk one side.

Baby overwhelmed by milk supply

If your let-down is so strong that the milk gushes into the baby's mouth and nearly chokes him, you'll find it helps if you collect this early milk in a sterilised container and allow your baby to continue feeding only when the milk has stopped flowing so exuberantly. If necessary you can give him the collected milk by spoon afterwards.

Babies who try to swallow quickly enough to cope with such an exuberant milk supply may swallow too much air with the milk and so develop colic or regurgitate more than usual after a feed. Some babies bring up almost a whole feed because of this. Expressing or just collecting the initial milk you let down as described above should get over the problem. If you simply allow the baby to bring up a whole feed and then feed him again, he'll certainly keep the milk down because the flow will be much slower and he won't swallow so much air, but your milk supply will increase because of the law of demand and supply and your let-down will subsequently work even better, so making the problem worse at the next feed. One way of overcoming the problem of *too much milk* is to give one breast per feed, letting the baby suck on the empty breast for comfort (see page 110). Give the other breast at the next feed. This allows the baby to suck for comfort without getting two breasts full of milk at each feed. Express some milk from the unused breast to keep you comfortable if necessary. See also pages 99 and 147.

Low birth weight

One of the most difficult feeding situations is when you have a low birth weight baby which has been born early (a *pre-term* or *premature* baby). About 7 per cent of all newborn babies are of low birth weight and two thirds of these are less than thirty-seven weeks old. Generally, the more immature the baby, the less likely there is to be a sucking reflex (see page 14) and the more perseverance is needed on your part to keep up your milk supply until your baby grows mature enough to suck.

Technically, a low birth weight baby is one weighing less than five and a half pounds (2,500 g), but even five- and six-pound babies may not feed as well as bigger ones. A pre-term baby weighing less than two or three pounds will not have a sucking reflex at all and will have to be tube fed. As he matures, the sucking reflex will gradually appear.

Occasionally, a baby may be smaller than expected from the length of the pregnancy: that is, 'small for gestational age' or 'small for dates', because he has been poorly nourished in the uterus. Some small-for-dates babies suck poorly and have a poorly coordinated swallowing reflex at first. They tend to have a lot of mucus, which makes them gag and regurgitate.

Your small-for-dates baby may have a sucking reflex in spite of weighing very little so it's worth asking the doctors looking after him whether you should try suckling, whatever his weight, unless you know that he is also very premature. These babies need frequent feeding from birth onwards. The nursing and medical staff will be concerned to see that they are kept warm and that your breast milk, whether given by breast or tube, is sufficient to prevent a low level of blood sugar from developing.

Premature and small-for-dates babies do best on breast milk. Indeed, many hospitals give them breast milk from a milk bank if their mothers don't want to give them their own milk though milk from his own mother is best for a pre-term baby, as its composition is tailored to his immaturity.

Breast milk from a mother of a premature baby has a raised concentration of protein, ionised calcium, chloride and immuno-globulin A and less lactose. Breast milk is important for the baby to have not only because of its specific nutritional composition but also because of its immunological advantages. The premature baby, even more than the full-term baby, needs the protection against infection and allergy that only breast milk can provide. What's more, the mother who breastfeeds her premature baby may find it easier to feel close to him. Bonding is often difficult amidst the mother–infant separation and the technical paraphernalia of a special care baby unit or an intensive care unit. There is still some medical controversy over what to feed very tiny premature babies with, but the balance of opinion seems to be swinging to the mother's own breast milk rather than cows' milk (or other) formula for the tiny baby well enough to take milk but not mature or well enough to suck. The breast milk is given by a fine tube (gavage or nasogastric tube) passed down the nose and back of the throat into the gullet and thence to the stomach. This tube stays in this position between feeds. Feeds are given down the tube frequently, perhaps hourly. Breast milk given in this way is usually best pumped from the mother's breasts with an electric pump, though it can be manually expressed. Hand expression takes longer and is not always as effective in producing milk as is a pump, but some mothers prefer it.

One recent study showed that greater volumes of milk could be produced by mothers of pre-term babies if they used an oxytocin nasal spray in each nostril just before they used the electric pump. The spraying was repeated just before pumping the second breast. Although your tiny baby won't need large volumes for some time, you need to empty your breasts as well as possible at short, regular intervals in order to stimulate a good milk supply. It's just as important to collect your milk soon after birth as it would be if you had a baby of normal size, and just as important to prevent problems such as engorgement.

Experience in one centre in the US shows that pre-term infants who receive sugar water and cows' milk formula complements *lose more weight* than those who are breastfed frequently at the breast and given nothing else.

Premature babies are nursed in incubators in special care baby units to keep them warm and to protect them from infection. This means that you will have to go to your baby when you want to see him, though someone else can collect your milk and take it to him. Physical contact is very important both for your baby and for the development of your mothering instinct, which isn't always spontaneous by any means. If the staff will let you, hold your baby as often as you can, or at least stroke him gently through the armholes in the incubator.

It's all too easy as the mother of a pre-term baby to take your cue from the nursing staff as to how to handle your baby. However, the nurses are expert at medical and nursing care and often don't have the time to mother their small charges. As a result, all too often neither the nurses nor the mother gives the baby the physical contact (cuddling, stroking and holding) and attention he needs. When the baby is taken home, if he is a first baby, he's likely to be looked after in the same limited-touch way that his mother learnt while he was in hospital. This will not only affect the way he develops but will also spoil the nature of the relationship between him and his mother.

Maybe this is partly why babies who were born pre-term tend to cry twice as much as full-term babies do. No one will laugh at you if you talk to your pre-term baby, if you spend time looking at him or if you ask to be allowed to do as many of the routine nursing jobs such as nappy changing as possible.

Even before your baby has grown mature enough to suck, hold him at your breast. When he seems ready to suck, offer your breast every so often. The nasogastric tube can stay in place. There is no need to give a rubber teat to test for his readiness to suck. At first he may not suck and you'll need to persevere for some days or perhaps even weeks, keeping your milk supply going in the meantime.

Many pre-term babies start to suck really strongly at the breast only at about the time they were originally expected to be born. The more immature they are when they begin sucking at the breast, the more tired breastfeeding will make them as it requires such a lot of effort. *Don't be surprised if your pre-term baby just licks your breast during the first few sessions, or if he seems to go to sleep for up to twenty minutes between bouts of two or three proper sucks.* He's just regaining his strength and as long as he's warmly wrapped up next to your warm body, he'll be all right. Change him from side to side every so often during a feeding session and be prepared for these sessions to last a long time. Not for your baby a ten minutes-a-side feed! Try getting your milk to let down before your baby starts sucking and don't be afraid to adjust your position until it's good. Try and fit in *at least* eight to ten breastfeeds a day for your premature baby. The normal full-term baby would have this sort of number of feeds and the pre-term baby, who is taking smaller feeds, needs at least the same number and ideally more in order to take sufficient milk. During the transitional period from full tube-feeding to full breast-feeding, you'll find it much easier if you can live in the hospital and be as near your baby as possible.

With enough support from the nursing staff and from your paediatrician, and with the knowledge that you couldn't do better for your pre-term baby than give him your milk, you'll cope. It's all too easy to get depressed over minor and unimportant fluctuations in the amount of milk you produce. Try to relax as you mother your baby in a very special way during this time. Talk if you can to other mothers breastfeeding premature babies. Some baby units have regular support group meetings for just this. If you have to return home without your baby, borrow an electric pump to use at home so that you can take your milk to the hospital each time you visit.

Collect your milk in *small* quantities. Liaise with your baby's nurses to find how much they are giving him down the tube at each feed. Amounts as small as 10 to 15 ml are normal for a baby just over two pounds. Close the bag tightly and label it with your name and date. You can keep it in the fridge for up to 48 to 72 hours; in the freezing compartment of your fridge for about two weeks; or in the deep freeze for several months.

Ideally it's best if your pre-term baby never has a bottle, even if he has to be nursed in an incubator for several weeks. With expert help, he should be able to progress from tube-feeding with breast milk, to part breastfeeding, to full breastfeeding. Once he gets used to feeding from a bottle, you'll have problems with getting him to suck effectively at the breast (see page 172) so ask the staff to avoid giving him one at all if possible.

A difficulty arises if your baby is kept in hospital and you go home, because although you can still provide breast milk for his feeds, you won't be able to be there to breastfeed him every time he needs a feed. It's sometimes possible in such circumstances for the baby to be given your milk by spoon, rather than by bottle. Ideally it's preferable for you to stay in hospital with your premature baby until he can come home too.

Breast milk banks

Milk is supplied to these banks by breastfeeding mothers with milk to spare and can be transported by road or rail if necessary to premature or sick babies in hospitals with no access to donated breast milk.

Donor mothers are screened carefully before their milk is accepted. Their medical history, blood tests and drug intake are noted. If the mother is taking any drugs, including nicotine (from smoking), alcohol, aspirin and the Pill, her milk is not accepted. Careful instructions are given to her about how to collect and store her milk. The milk is cultured to make sure the bacteria count is low enough, pasteurised if necessary and frozen for a maximum of six months. The pasteurisation is best done by the 'flash' method to decrease the inactivation of antibodies and enzymes. Ideally, donated breast milk is used without being sterilised at all. Pasteurisation destroys lipase. Babies fed on pasteurised milk put on less weight than those given 'raw' breast milk, as lipase is necessary for the absorption of fat. Live cells are also destroyed.

Breast milk from these banks has helped save the lives of many sick or tiny babies whose own mothers could not or would not feed them themselves.

If you have milk to spare and are prepared to donate it to other babies, mention this to your doctor, local hospital, National

Childbirth Trust teacher or breastfeeding counsellor, or La Leche League leader. They will advise you what to do.

The baby with teeth

Some babies are actually born with one or two teeth, though most don't get a tooth for the first six months at least. There is no reason why teeth should interfere with breastfeeding as the baby's gums are not used for feeding: the pressure comes from the tongue below and the palate above.

Your baby may, however, try the odd bite when he's older and will be very interested in your reaction. It's best to say 'no' firmly and gently take him off the breast. If you smile, he may think you like it and do it again! Some babies bite only towards the end of a feed and this is easily handled. Simply take him off the breast before he starts to bite; you'll soon get to know when he's about to do it.

Some mothers have found a rubber nipple shield useful if their baby likes to bite.

Finally, remember that some babies bite from frustration if the breast is too full or if there is not enough milk. You can cope with this sort of biting by dealing with the underlying problem.

13 Some special situations

Baby ill or in hospital

Unless your baby is so ill that he is not allowed any milk, he'll do better with *your* milk than with any other and will make a faster recovery after such illnesses as gastroenteritis if his bowel doesn't have to cope with cows' milk formula.

If he has to go into hospital, the ideal is for you to go too so you can be near him to comfort and support him emotionally and also to feed him. If you can spend the day with him but can't stay at night, then leave as much expressed or pumped milk as you can for the nurses to give him from a spoon (or from a bottle if he is so experienced at breastfeeding that it's unlikely that he'll learn to prefer a bottle).

If you can visit only infrequently you may need to bring enough milk for several days. You'll need patience to express or pump your breasts frequently (more often than your baby usually feeds) day after day but it can be done and is easiest if you can borrow an electric breast pump to use at home.

When your baby has his immunisations he may go off his milk and be more fussy than usual for about twenty-four hours. If you're getting over-full because he's not sucking well, simply express a little milk every so often. You'll need to do this whenever he wants less milk for a day or two when he's feeling unwell for some reason.

Baby jaundiced

There are many causes of jaundice (yellow colouring of the skin caused by high levels of the yellow pigment bilirubin in the blood) in the first few weeks of life, ranging from 'physiological' jaundice which many babies get, to abnormal jaundice from infection, a congenital defect, drugs, or ABO or rhesus blood group incompatibility, which can be serious if not treated adequately. The diagnosis depends on the time of onset of the jaundice and on the results of the blood tests.

Only a few full-term babies with jaundice need treatment and the type of treatment given depends on the type of jaundice and on the level of bilirubin in the baby's blood. Blood tests are taken frequently to see whether the bilirubin level is rising or falling. Jaundice is a common occurrence in both breast- and bottle-fed babies.

Some experts consider that physiological jaundice (following the breakdown of red blood cells in the newborn baby) may be increased if a breastfed baby is not fed soon after birth and thereafter on a frequent and unrestricted basis. This sort of jaundice appears on the second to fourth day of life and usually goes in about a week. Colostrum helps the baby's bowel get rid of meconium – the first bowel motions which contain a lot of bilirubin that if not quickly excreted can be reabsorbed into the baby's bloodstream. Water given as an extra has been shown not to be helpful and may also interfere with the mother's milk supply as her baby will demand fewer feeds at the breast if his tummy is filled with water. Any baby, including a jaundiced baby, does best with a good milk supply. This is most likely to happen if breastfeeding is done frequently and on an unrestricted basis. If your jaundiced baby is given drinks of water in hospital, do be sure to stimulate your milk supply by hand expression after or even between feeds to make up for the reduction in sucking from your baby whose thirst is slaked with water.

Babies with abnormal jaundice often look yellow at birth or within the first twenty-four hours afterwards. Whatever other treatment may be necessary for these babies, they should be breastfed early, frequently and on an unrestricted basis for the same reasons as outlined above.

Babies with moderately raised levels of bilirubin are often treated by phototherapy (light therapy) by being placed uncovered in a cot sixteen inches beneath a daylight fluorescent tube with their eyes covered to protect them. One big snag with this is that it may interfere with unrestricted breastfeeding and consequently the mother's milk supply may not increase as fast as it should. However, there's no reason why you shouldn't take your baby from under the light and feed him two-hourly (or more often if he demands it). If your baby is otherwise well, your paediatrician may agree to your taking your baby home because there you can give him daylight photo-therapy if you keep him uncovered by a window in strong daylight. Beware of sunburn and don't let him get too cold or hot. You'll be told to bring him back to the hospital for blood tests so that the bilirubin level can be observed. The advantage of taking your baby home is that you can breastfeed much more easily there.

Pre-term babies are affected adversely by lower raised levels of bilirubin than are full term ones, so any necessary treatment will be started sooner. Breastfeeding is just as important for these babies and skilled help and support from the nursery staff will make all the difference to you.

Breast milk jaundice

Very rarely a baby develops jaundice from breast milk. Although this sort of jaundice would disappear within three to seven days if he were taken off the breast, it is necessary to interrupt breastfeeding only if the levels of bilirubin in his blood rise to unacceptably high levels. If your baby's bilirubin level rises too high, your paediatrician will advise you to interrupt breastfeeding for a short time. There is some difference of opinion as to how long this should be, but one expert says it only needs to be as short as twelve hours. If at the end of this time the bilirubin level has fallen significantly (by more than 2 mg/100ml), breastfeeding can be resumed. Usually the bilirubin level then rises slightly before falling slowly and steadily. If it rises again later, breastfeeding should again be interrupted. If the bilirubin level doesn't fall significantly after a twelve-hour break, the break should be extended by six to twelve hours, measuring the bilirubin level every four to six hours. Clearly if the level rises during the breaks from breastfeeding, the jaundice is not due to breast milk. While your baby is off breast milk, keep your milk supply going by expressing or pumping more frequently than your baby would have been fed, and discard your milk until your baby can again be breastfed. Your baby can be given donated breast milk or cows' milk formula in the interval.

The cause of breast milk jaundice has yet to be fully elucidated, but is thought to be due to a particular chemical in the milk which interferes with the metabolism of bilirubin in the baby, causing high levels of bilirubin in the blood. Apart from this particular type of jaundice, jaundice is equally likely to occur in breast- and bottle-fed babies. It is, of course, important for an accurate diagnosis to be made so as to rule out any more serious causes of the jaundice. Breast milk jaundice tends to appear towards the end of the first week of life, is worst during the second to third week and lasts from three weeks to two months.

Rhesus antibodies

Many mothers who know they have rhesus antibodies in their blood worry that, if they breastfeed, these antibodies may be passed to the baby via the milk. Rhesus antibodies are present in breast milk if they are present in the mother's blood but they have no effect on the baby because they are inactivated in his gut. It is therefore quite safe to breastfeed your rhesus positive baby if you are rhesus negative and have rhesus antibodies, even if he is jaundiced. Indeed, it's the best way to feed these babies, according to several studies. It is also quite safe to breastfeed after having an injection of anti-D immunoglobulin.

The baby with a cleft lip and/or palate

The initial shock of discovering that your baby has a cleft lip, with or without a cleft palate, may make you reluctant to breastfeed. If you can get over this initial feeling of disappointment, you'll remember that you never see older children walking around with any noticeable deformity of their lips. The plastic surgery available today is so good that the defect can be almost perfectly repaired.

A cleft lip by itself needn't interfere with breastfeeding. Some milk may leak out around the cleft but you should soon learn how to press the lip around your breast to form a seal. Your baby will be able to suck (unless the cleft is exceptionally severe) and also to milk the breast.

Many units are now repairing cleft lips within two days of birth, though others still wait the traditional three months or so before operating. Early surgery is by far the best from the feeding point of view, as not only does it make feeding easier for the baby but it also makes the mother feel emotionally more inclined to breastfeed.

Different surgeons advise waiting for different lengths of time before the baby is allowed to suck after a cleft lip repair. Because of the danger of the scar splitting open, some suggest waiting for three to four weeks, while others allow sucking at ten days and yet others immediately after surgery. From both the mother's and the baby's points of view, the sooner feeding is started, the better, but obviously the healing of the scar takes priority. While you are waiting to resume breastfeeding after the surgery, keep your milk supply going by frequent and regular expression or pumping, preferably with an electric pump. Your milk can be given to your baby by a spoon.

If it's decided to postpone the operation for several months, you'll need a lot of patience while feeding, as babies with a cleft lip tend to take a long time over their feeds.

If your baby has a severe cleft lip and you find it impossible to breastfeed, you can still give him your milk from a specially shaped spoon or a bottle with an adapted teat. Ask your paediatrician about these.

A baby with a cleft palate can't suck the nipple and areola because air is drawn in from the nose when he tries to suck. You can make up for the loss of suction by holding your nipple and areola in his mouth all the time he feeds, using a cigarette hold. Once the breast is held in place like this, the baby will be able to milk it satisfactorily with practice. You may find a Lact-aid useful while your baby is learning to milk your breast and this will avoid confusing him with a bottle.

It's been noticed that breast milk doesn't irritate the mucous membranes of the nose of a baby with a cleft palate, unlike cows' milk formula. Because such babies are particularly prone to middle ear infection (otitis media) this is a point in favour of breastfeeding, which is associated with less otitis media than is bottle-feeding. Most mothers find it is better to breastfeed their baby with a cleft palate in a relatively upright position to minimise the chance of milk going into the nose.

A dental plate (sometimes called a 'pre-surgical appliance' or 'feeding plate') can be made for a baby with a cleft palate for use until the cleft is repaired, usually after the baby is a year old. Each plastic plate is individually made from impressions taken of the palate. It can be inserted as early as three days after birth and not only helps the baby to feed satisfactorily but also improves the alignment of the dental arches. Plates are made routinely at some hospitals and used for severe clefts in others.

The mentally handicapped baby

There is every reason why you should breastfeed your mentally handicapped baby. He will get the same benefits from being breastfed as any other baby and it will help cement the bond between you.

One mother of a baby with Down's syndrome (mongolism) commented 'I'm sure that breastfeeding and the closeness that comes with it helped me to love and accept him just as he was.' Babies with this condition are more prone to infection, particularly respiratory infection, than other babies, so the immunity provided by breast milk is especially valuable for them.

Some of these babies feed rather apathetically because of muscle weakness, a poor sucking reflex or general sleepiness and so take a long time over their feeds, but bottle-feeding is just as time-consuming. With patience you'll succeed and you'll be sure you're doing the best for your baby. Just as with any baby, avoid using a bottle because learning to bottle-suck will interfere with his learning to suck at the breast. If your baby is too tired to suck for long, express some milk and give it to him via a dropper or a spoon. You may need to encourage your baby to suck by giving him lots of skin contact, starting your let-down reflex before you put him to the breast, or expressing a few drops of your milk into his mouth, for instance. Try to put him to your breast before he has to cry, to avoid tiring him. If he is so sleepy that he doesn't wake very often, wake him up for a feed every two hours or so if necessary.

Many women with handicapped babies feel that they deserve every possible help and chance in life and that breastfeeding is the best starting point.

Failure to thrive (see also page 132)

The term 'failure to thrive' simply means that *a baby isn't growing as he should*. There are arbitrary definitions to guide doctors who see babies who aren't gaining weight normally, but each baby has to be assessed as an individual. For practical purposes, if a baby continues to lose weight after ten days of life, if he hasn't regained his birth weight by three weeks, or if he gains weight at a rate below the tenth percentile on the percentile chart after he is one month old, this will alert the doctor to the fact that all may not be well.

There are many reasons why a breastfed baby may not be growing optimally. He may not be drinking enough milk (because of poor sucking or swallowing, or infrequent, short feeds); he may be losing nutrients (because of malabsorption, diarrhoea or vomiting); he may have an infection (for example in the urinary tract); or he may have especially high energy needs which are not being met (for example, the baby who is small-for-dates or has a congenital heart disease). His mother may not be producing enough milk (because of poor diet, illness or exhaustion) or she may not be letting her milk down (for psychosocial reasons, because she's a heavy smoker or drinker, or because of certain drugs). Eventually a poor let-down leads to poor production. Several problems may be combined, which is why the doctor will take a careful and complete medical, social and dietary history, examine the baby thoroughly, look at the mother's breasts, watch the baby being fed and arrange for various laboratory tests.

The most common cause of failure to thrive is simply that the baby isn't getting enough milk because he isn't being put to the breast often enough or for long enough. The consequently diminished milk supply is easily put right once the mother realises the problem. *A more difficult problem is if the baby isn't sucking and milking the breast well.*

Certain medical conditions can reduce the strength of the baby's sucking and milking action, including Down's syndrome (mongolism), trisomy 13-15 (another congenital abnormality), kernicterus (following severe untreated jaundice), infantile spinal muscular atrophy, congenital muscular dystrophy, neonatal myasthenia gravis, infections of the central nervous system, and hypothyroidism. These conditions are uncommon and you can leave it to your paediatrician to diagnose them.

More common medical reasons for poor sucking and milking by the baby include the effect on the baby of drugs given to the mother in labour which passed across the placenta before the baby was born (these drugs can take a long time to disappear from the baby's body), immaturity of the baby following a pre-term birth, and the after effects of a poor oxygen supply to the baby during labour.

Other medical conditions can affect the efficiency of a baby's sucking and milking action, including mechanical factors such as a large tongue, cleft lip, and certain congenital abnormalities of the gums and jaws. Finally, the baby may have difficulty in swallowing for a variety of reasons including cleft palate, inflammation following intubation for breathing difficulties at birth, and a congenitally small lower jaw. If swallowing is difficult, the baby automatically milks the breast poorly.

Some of these conditions, for example hypothyroidism and infections of the central nervous system, are relatively easily treatable and the baby's sucking and milking action will improve after treatment. Others improve spontaneously. With untreatable or less easily treatable conditions, the baby will have to be helped a lot if breastfeeding is to be successful.

Apart from medical reasons for a poor sucking and milking action, a baby may suck poorly because he is tired, jaundiced, or full (see page 171). There may be straightforward practical problems such as poor positioning at the breast (see page 159), poorly protractile nipples (see page 159) or engorgement (see page 154).

Commonly, a baby may have been given one or more bottles of cows' milk formula even though his mother is supposed to be breastfeeding. While such an action may be well meant, it can play havoc with breastfeeding simply because it is so easy for a baby to bottle-suck and often, subsequently, so difficult for him to learn how to breastfeed (see page 172).

The usual story of a baby with a poor sucking, milking or swallowing action who is failing to gain enough weight in spite of his mother knowing all about unrestricted breastfeeding is that he is at the breast very frequently, sometimes hourly or even more or less non-stop day and night. Some babies don't seem interested in feeding; they are 'happy to starve' and may sleep for very long periods. The mother is often tired out and desperate for help. The baby has probably only been getting foremilk because he hasn't been stimulating the breast well enough with his poor suck to let the hindmilk down. To get a large enough volume of milk, he has to suck very often but because foremilk is relatively low in calories, he doesn't put on enough weight. Because a poor let-down eventually leads to a lowered milk production, continuing like this is doomed to failure.

Instead of initiating the let-down of his mother's milk by sucking with a rapid fluttering movement, then sucking slowly and swallowing after each suck, then waiting for a while before starting the whole process again, up to eight times in one session, the baby with sucking and milking problems may use only a rapid fluttering movement with little swallowing. Often the baby swallows for the first five minutes when getting the foremilk and then no more. A good way of telling whether a baby is swallowing is to watch for movements in front of his ear, and to listen. He may sleep for twenty minutes or so between bouts of only two or three sucks, and he may keep his eyes closed for much of the time. You may also notice that occasionally his *cheeks are hollowed by being sucked in*. This is caused by tongue sucking: if you pull his lower lip down you'll see that his tongue is above the nipple instead of below it. Sometimes *the tongue is stuck out* (tongue 'thrusting') and this makes the baby come off the breast. *The first thing to do is to find out why the baby is having trouble in sucking, milking or swallowing and if possible to put it right*. If there is no apparent reason, if the cause is untreatable, or even if it has been treated successfully, there are several things that can be tried to help a baby get the milk from his mother.

1 *Check the position of the baby and the mother.* (Baby's body facing mother's; baby's head resting on her arm, with the hand of her arm palm down: if the hand is palm up, the baby may drop off the breast; baby shouldn't be dragging the nipple up or down – cushions may help get him at the right height; mother shouldn't be holding the baby's head; baby's bottom should be close to mother).

2 *Check that the nipple and areola are being offered attractively.* (Soften the breast first if full of milk by expressing a little; encourage the nipple to erect; rub some milk on to the nipple so that the baby can smell and taste it straight away; get the let-down working before the baby goes to the breast or set up the Lact-aid, if you are using one, so that the milk flows immediately so as to encourage the

baby; either hold the breast as if on a shelf, with your opposite hand supporting it from below, or use a cigarette hold to make a 'biscuit' of the nipple and areola in such a way that the 'biscuit' is in parallel with the baby's mouth. Some experienced counsellors say that the 'shelf support' works best for a baby with sucking and milking difficulties; try tickling the baby's lips with the nipple and when he opens his mouth, draw him closer to the breast).

3 *Change sides as soon as he stops swallowing* (often every five minutes or so) during a feed. This is called switch nursing (or the 'burp and switch technique'), encourages the baby to suck better and also stimulates the let-down. As you are changing him over, encourage him to wake up if he's sleepy by burping him (bending him at the waist is a good way).

4 Experiment to see if the baby takes the breast better if the room is *quiet*, if he is *tightly wrapped* or if he is *unwrapped and not too warm*. Try breastfeeding with you and him both *naked* to see if the skin contact stimulates him to suck better. *Talk or sing or jiggle him* gently to rouse him. *Praise him* after a good sucking session: even a young baby may respond by doing it again.

5 As the baby's sucking and milking are improved by 1 to 4 above, don't forget to wake him for feeds if he's been in the habit of sleeping for long periods. *Your milk supply needs stimulating* now and it's no good getting him to suck properly if there's no milk for him. While his improved sucking will in itself increase your milk supply, it needs to be combined with reasonably frequent, unrestricted feeds, with no long gaps between them. Aim at first for no more than two hours between feeds (from the start of one to the start of the next) during the day, and three hours at night, though if your baby wants more, of course put him to the breast (see page 135).

6 *Aim for realistic goals as far as weight goes.* If your baby has been putting on no weight, then a gain of two ounces in the next week is very good. If he's been losing, to stay still is good.

7 If you can't improve your baby's sucking and milking actions, try

using a *Lact-aid* filled with milk you've expressed or pumped after each feed. Your baby will be getting your milk at your breast. Once you've got used to it, a Lact-aid is as easy to sterilise and fill as a bottle. A Lact-aid is also useful immediately if your paediatrician says that the baby needs extra milk. If you can't produce enough milk to put in it, use cows' milk formula or donated breast milk and increase your milk supply by expressing or pumping regularly and frequently. As a last resort, *bottle-feed your baby with your expressed or pumped milk*.

Rare illnesses

Galactosaemia is an inborn condition caused by an enzyme deficiency which can sometimes be fatal if the baby is not put on a lactose- (milk sugar-) free diet. There is no alternative but to wean your baby at once.

Certain other 'inborn errors of metabolism', for example phenylketonuria, may be diagnosed soon after birth. A combination of breastfeeding plus a special formula milk is best for these babies. Careful monitoring of certain metabolites in the baby is usually necessary.

Mother ill

If you are acutely *ill* at home and have to be in bed, you'll need someone to look after you and the baby and bring the baby to you when he is ready for a feed, assuming you are too unwell to have him in bed with you or in a cot by your bed. If you have to go into hospital, you may be able to take the baby with you, but this will depend on what is wrong with you and on the hospital's rules and facilities. If you can't have your baby with you, then it may be possible for someone to bring him to you for feeds, though this entails a lot of work and means that you'll need to be in a hospital close to your home.

Yet another way of carrying on breastfeeding if you're in hospital is to express or pump milk and send it home for the baby. It should be stored in a refrigerator until collected by a friend or relative to be given to the baby by spoon.

There are a few illnesses which actually rule out breastfeeding. Others do so, perhaps temporarily, because of the drugs used to treat them. If you have a *chronic illness* such as severe asthma or kidney disease, you may feel so permanently tired and run down that you can't cope with nursing your baby as well. Some mothers manage, though, and find that the feeding times make them rest and so tire them less than bottle-feeding would.

Diabetes

Diabetes certainly is a common condition, affecting about 2 per cent of the population, but because so few diabetic women choose to breastfeed, research into the effects on a diabetic mother and her baby is scanty. In one American study, seventeen breastfeeding, insulin-dependent diabetic mothers were followed, fourteen of whom fed their babies for more than nine months. Several useful tips came out of their experiences. High motivation and unusual support from family, friends and health professionals meant that all these women were able to breastfeed successfully. Care is especially necessary if baby and mother are separated after delivery. Frequent expression of milk or, preferably, visits to the baby for him to be cuddled and put to the breast are essential to work up the milk supply.

About five to seven hours after delivery there is an increased risk of the mother's blood sugar becoming too low (hypoglycaemia) since the loss of the hormone placental lactogen is accompanied by an increased sensitivity to insulin. This happens whether or not a mother is breastfeeding, and as soon as diet-insulin-exercise adjustments are made, the blood sugar stabilises. Most mothers find that during the first four to six weeks their insulin requirement is less than before they became pregnant. Breastfeeding itself may reduce the insulin requirement for longer than this period. Four women in the survey, however, needed more insulin during the first three months after delivery than before they became pregnant, probably because they were eating more and exercising less.

Hypoglycaemic (insulin) reactions cause the release of adrenalin which decreases the blood flow through the arteries in the breasts and can also inhibit the let-down reflex. Traces of insulin and adrenalin pass into the milk but are inactivated by the baby's digestive enzymes.

Infections should always be treated quickly in diabetics and the antibiotic chosen must be safe for the breastfed baby. Diabetic women are more prone to monilial ('thrush') infection of the vagina which can spread to affect the nipples.

Breastfed babies may suddenly want either more or less frequent feeds, perhaps because of illness or a growth spurt. This can cause unexpectedly low or high blood sugar levels in diabetic mothers which can be compensated for by adjusting the diet, exercise and insulin dose.

Some doctors find that their diabetic patients are more stable when breastfeeding than they were before. Doctors who deal a lot with diabetic mothers find that they seem to have more difficulty in producing milk than do non-diabetic women but this is only a generalisation and many diabetic mothers feed perfectly satisfactorily.

Pulmonary tuberculosis

If you have had pulmonary tuberculosis and have been free from the disease for two years, you can feed your baby quite safely.

If a mother has had active pulmonary tuberculosis during pregnancy, with a positive tuberculin test, a positive chest X-ray and bacteriologically positive sputum or gastric washings, and if her treatment (with 'triple' therapy: three drugs) was begun *at least a week before her baby was born*, then she needn't be separated from her baby and she can safely breastfeed him *provided he is also treated with isoniazid*. If a mother is bacteriologically negative, then her baby can be breastfed even if her treatment has only just begun, provided he too is treated with isoniazid (in a smaller dose than for the baby whose mother is bacteriologically positive). It is important that the baby doesn't get too much isoniazid because he'll be getting some in the breast milk as well, so some experts suggest that liver function should be monitored by serial blood tests. (Overdosage can cause peripheral neuritis.) Because one of the commonly used drugs in the 'triple' therapy, para-aminosalicylic acid (PAS), is not recommended for babies (though it's not known for sure how much gets through into breast milk), the mother may be given streptomycin or kanamycin instead. If other drugs are used, special precautions may be advisable.

If a breastfeeding mother contracts active, bacteriologically positive tuberculosis, a period of separation from her baby may be recommended for safety while drug treatment is begun and until her sputum and gastric washings are negative on culture. If her milk is not infected, it is reasonable for her to express or pump it for it to be given to the baby by spoon. Usually she can be rendered non-infectious within a very short time. It could be argued that if the mother and baby have been together anyway before the tuberculosis in the mother was diagnosed, then there is no point in separating them, but because complications of tuberculosis are more hazardous in the newborn period, it is worth taking every precaution to reduce the baby's chance of contracting the disease. There is some controversy over the medical management of the breastfeeding mother with tuberculosis and her baby in developed countries. In certain developing countries and among certain isolated peoples such as some American Indians, it is virtually always safer to leave the mother and baby together than to separate them, simply because breastfeeding is usually so much safer for the baby than bottle-feeding, given the lack of money to buy cows' milk formula powder, the lack of bottle sterilisation facilities and the high risk of infection. The risk of unmonitored drug toxicity is relatively unimportant in such circumstances. These breastfed babies should be carefully treated with isoniazid, however, and vaccinated with a special type of BCG vaccine (isoniazid-resistant vaccine). The mother's active tuberculosis needs thorough treatment at the same time.

Other problems

Several other infections may temporarily produce problems for the breastfeeding mother, but in no case is it necessary to dry up the milk. If it seems advisable that the baby shouldn't drink his mother's milk for some reason, then she should keep her milk supply going by frequent expression or pumping and discard the milk. As soon as the baby is allowed her breast milk again, she'll then have no problems with a decreased milk supply. She'll also avoid the pain of engorgement at the time when she's probably not feeling too well anyway. If *gonorrhoea* is diagnosed at the time of delivery, no breast milk should be given the baby and there should be no contact between the baby and the mother until twenty-four hours after drug treatment has been begun.

Infectious syphilitic skin on the breasts means that the baby shouldn't be fed at the breast, but the milk can usually be expressed or pumped and given to him. The mother with *leprosy* is advised not to hold her baby except to breastfeed him, as breastfeeding is recognised as being valuable enough to outweigh any possible dangers. Both mother and baby are given drug treatment.

Mothers with *severe deficiency of vitamin B₁* (thiamine) causing the disease beri-beri should not breastfeed their babies as toxic substances are present in the milk. This condition is thankfully not seen in the western world, though it is still said to exist in parts of China.

Infertility caused by *hyperprolactinaemia* can be successfully treated with a drug called bromocriptine. This lowers the blood prolactin level and enables conception to occur. Once you've got your baby, though, the drug can't be used to keep the prolactin low if you want to breastfeed, because it dries the milk up!

Because breastfeeding raises the blood prolactin level further, women may be discouraged from doing it for two reasons. First there seems to be five times the risk of getting a breast abscess and, second, a sizeable proportion of women with this condition have a tumour of the pituitary gland. Raising the prolactin level by breastfeeding could lead to an increase in the size of such a tumour. Because of the position of the tumour, enlargement can lead to visual disturbances, including blindness.

If the raised prolactin levels of pregnancy have not already led to an increase in size of a woman's tumour (as gauged by visual field measurement and special X-rays), and if she wants to breastfeed, a woman could have regular checks of her visual field and regular X-rays so that she could stop breastfeeding at the first suspicion of any increase in tumour size. These tests are, however, time-consuming and expensive.

Caesarean section

Many babies today are born by Caesarean section (more than a half in some US hospitals). After this operation there is no reason why you shouldn't breastfeed but you'll need to be extra determined in the first week or so. There are two main problems. First, you're likely to have a certain amount of abdominal pain and discomfort because a Caesarean section is a serious abdominal operation. This discomfort may make you feel very unmotherly towards your baby. If you are to get your milk supply going well, it's best to feed your baby frequently by day and night, just as you would had you had a normal delivery. It's really just as easy to feed the baby as it is to express or pump your milk and you are less likely to have the added problems of engorgement and sore nipples if you feed on demand from the beginning. You'll also prevent your baby from having cows' milk formula. Of course, you may not be able to feed your baby immediately after delivery if you have had a general anaesthetic but as soon as you are awake or well enough ask for your baby to be brought to you for a feed, even if he is asleep. More Caesarean sections are being performed today under epidural anaesthesia which means that breastfeeding gets off to a better start.

The second problem is also related to your operation. You'll find it uncomfortable to feed in the normal sitting position with the baby on your lap. Enlist the help of a nurse at each feed time to position the baby next to you as you are lying down on one side in bed. When the time comes to change breasts, ring for a nurse to help you turn over and bring the baby to your other side.

If you have a horizontal scar, you can try sitting up, lying the baby on a pillow with his head facing the breast and his legs tucked under your arm on that side. Alternatively, with you sitting up, lie him on a pillow at your side with his legs across your thighs and support his head either with another pillow at the correct height or with your arm, in turn supported by a pillow. The point of all these positions is to take the weight of the baby off your abdomen and to avoid the strain on your abdominal muscles of holding the baby to your breast. Sit straight to avoid straining your abdomen.

By the end of the first week you should be feeling very much better and will be able to carry on just like any other breastfeeding mother.

If your Caesarean baby is nursed in an incubator after delivery and isn't allowed to come to you for feeds, express or pump your colostrum (and milk when it comes in). The nurses will give the breast milk feeds by tube or spoon, depending on the state of the baby, until you can go to him. Don't be alarmed by the small amounts of colostrum – remember there isn't much in the first day or so – but remember the special importance of colostrum to your baby.

A Caesarean section, especially if unplanned, can undermine a mother's opinion of herself. If she is helped to breastfeed her baby, she may think better of her capabilities as a woman. Breastfeeding is helpful to postoperative recovery because the production of oxytocin assists the uterus to return to its former size. A Caesarean section leaves some mothers feeling very tired for some time and it's important that they get enough rest. This doesn't mean that nights must be unbroken, with the baby given a bottle by the nursing staff, but that between feeds the day shouldn't be crammed full of activity on the ward or at home, but should allow ample time to sleep or catnap. Pain-killers may well be necessary especially in the first day or two because a Caesarean section scar can be painful while healing, especially when coughing. Many women need strong pain relief but simple drugs such as aspirin or codeine are quite suitable for others.

Toxaemia

Severe toxaemia can present initial problems with breastfeeding for several reasons: the baby may be pre-term or small-for-dates and hence may be nursed in an incubator; the mother may still be at risk of having convulsions and her treatment will include drugs to lower her blood pressure, sedation, bed rest and being nursed in a darkened room. Most mothers recover within 24 to 48 hours after delivery. How breastfeeding is managed depends on all these factors and each mother and baby pair must be considered separately. If the baby cannot be put to the breast, or if early feeds are unsuccessful and therefore stressful to the mother, expressing or pumping her milk will be considered. Expert nursing care is necessary to make either as easy and stress-free as possible for her. Some doctors consider that the stress and stimulation involved in pumping or expressing is too risky for the mother who may have an eclamptic fit, and are unhappy anyway about the possible accumulation of the mother's sedatives (usually phenobarbitone) and other drugs in the baby having breast milk. Points to consider, however, are that the stress factor in having engorged, unemptied breasts may be considerable in itself; that the mother may be anxious about her baby not being breastfed, unless she is extremely heavily sedated; and that the drugs normally given to the mother have not been shown (in the relatively small numbers studied) to be dangerous to breastfed babies, though care must be taken to ensure that the breastfed baby (especially if ill or pre-term) is not being 'depressed' by the accumulation of large doses of phenobarbitone.

If you are advised not to breastfeed and not to pump or express either, don't worry, because it's possible for you to get your milk supply back later when you are well. If your doctor is reluctant for your milk to be given to your baby because of high drug levels, you may be able (or the nurses may be able) to keep your milk supply going and the milk can be discarded until your medication level is reduced.

Drug treatment

Virtually every drug a mother takes will pass into her breast milk, though some reach much higher concentrations than others. Many drugs are harmless to the breastfed baby however high the concentration in the milk, while others may be potentially harmful even in tiny amounts, either because of known side-effects which affect adults as well, or because they have a different action in a young baby.

Some drugs can cause the development of sensitivity or allergy which may be dangerous when repeated doses are taken.

Knowledge of the effects of many drugs on the breastfed baby is far from complete because of the difficulty in doing drug trials in breastfeeding mothers. These are difficult because so few breastfeeding mothers are actually taking any one drug and it would be wrong to experiment by giving them potentially harmful drugs. There is also the very real difficulty of measuring the levels of drugs in milk and finally there's a general lack of interest in the whole subject, especially since the numbers of breastfeeding mothers fell over the very years that drug treatment increased.

Ideally, a breastfeeding mother should not take any drugs. However, this is obviously the counsel of perfection and there may be times when drugs will be life-saving and she'll have to take them. If they happen to be dangerous for the baby, then she'll have to wean, if only temporarily. There are other drugs which are not life-saving to the mother but are very useful in treating some illnesses. If the particular drug suggested is not safe for the breastfed baby, there is often an alternative which is. Occasionally, the known risks are so low that the mother and her doctor will feel justified in her carrying on with breastfeeding while she's taking the drug.

Rather than list the many drugs known to be safe to the breastfed infant, we'll mention the ones that are known to be *either unsafe or better avoided*. If you have any doubts at all, ask your doctor: he can contact the manufacturer of the drug for more details if necessary.

Side-effects of drugs in the breastfed baby
Anti-infective drugs
Chloramphenicol May harm the bone marrow. It may also cause refusal of the breast, sleepiness during feeds and vomiting after. Avoid while breastfeeding a baby under four weeks old.

Sulphonamides. If a baby is jaundiced, sulphonamides in breast milk may increase the jaundice. However, if there is only a trace of jaundice, the risk is negligible. Cautious use and careful observation are suggested if the baby is under one month old. Haemolytic anaemia has been reported in one G6PD deficient baby (a rare enzyme deficiency). Can cause a rash.

Tetracyclines Theoretically cause mottling of a baby's developing teeth, though probably bound by calcium in breast milk, which retards absorption. Two authors recommend their avoidance by breastfeeding mothers.

Penicillins Appear in trace amounts in breast milk and can theoretically cause allergic sensitisation. Resulting levels in the baby are not high enough to treat infection. An alternative antibiotic should ideally be used, though this may not always be possible.

Metronidazole According to the manufacturer, the traces excreted in breast milk are harmless. Although carcinogenicity was reported in mice given this drug, this is not considered relevant to the breastfed baby now. However, because of the slight risk of a blood dyscrasia, or of decreased appetite, vomiting and diarrhoea if high doses are used, it is sensible to use an alternative drug to treat trichomonas infection in the mother.

Nalidixic acid One case of haemolytic anemia has been reported in a baby whose mother was also taking amylobarbitone. It has also caused raised intracranial pressure. Use with caution only if absolutely necessary and observe the baby carefully.

Nitrofurantoin The level in breast milk is not pharmacologically significant, but caution is advised in G6PD-deficient babies.

Novobiocin Not recommended for breastfeeding mothers because of the possibility of neonatal jaundice.

Anticoagulants

Bleeding episodes have occurred after surgery or trauma in babies. Warfarin however is suitable for a breastfeeding mother, as is heparin. Other drugs should be used with caution or substituted where possible with warfarin or heparin.

Cytotoxic (anti-cancer) drugs Breastfeeding is generally contra-indicated though methotrexate and busulphan seem to present little hazard.

Anti-thyroid drugs

These may cause goitre in the baby which can be treated by giving him thyroxine. However, some also have the rare side-effect of causing a potentially fatal blood disorder. One study concludes that they are not absolutely contra-indicated provided the dose is small and that the circulating thyroid hormones of the baby are closely monitored. The authors felt that propylthiouracil was the preferred drug for a breastfeeding mother. Iodides (found in some cough medicines and sometimes used to treat hyperthyroidism) may suppress the baby's thyroid activity and cause goitre. They can also sensitise the baby's thyroid gland to lithium, chlorpromazine and methylxanthines.

Central nervous system drugs

Alcohol Amounts of alcohol large enough to make you 'tipsy' have been shown to reduce oxytocin levels and so hinder breastfeeding.

It can cause intoxication in the baby if large enough amounts are taken. Doses higher than 1 g/kg of the mother's weight can inhibit the let-down reflex, while doses higher than 2 g/kg probably block it completely.

Amantadine Contra-indicated in the breastfeeding mother, according to the manufacturers, as it may cause vomiting, urinary retention and rashes in the baby.

Barbiturates Can cause drowsiness and may also stimulate the metabolism of other drugs taken by the mother. One case of cyanosis ('blue baby') due to methaemoglobinaemia occurred in a baby whose mother was also taking phenytoin.

Bromide Usually causes drowsiness and may cause a rash.

Cannabis Animal studies have shown that brain cells can be damaged in newborn sucklings. Impairment of DNA and RNA formation by cannabis has been described. Also, prolactin levels in the mother are lowered.

Carbamazepine Not advised by the manufacturer if used in high doses or in combination with other anti-epileptics, as there is a structural likeness to the tricyclic anti-depressants which are not metabolised in the young baby. However, no side-effects have actually been reported in the baby whose mother is taking the drug alone.

Chloral hydrate Can cause drowsiness in a baby.

Chloroform Has been reported to cause deep sleep in babies.

Diazepam One report of lethargy and weight loss. The levels may build up in the baby's body and increase physiological jaundice. High doses should be used with caution in the breastfeeding mother.

Dichloralphenazone Causes slight drowsiness.

Heroin Can cause addiction in babies.

Lithium The baby should be carefully monitored for signs of lithium toxicity, including lethargy and floppiness.

Morphine Significant amounts may be excreted in the milk of addicts.

Phenytoin Many mothers have breastfed their babies while taking phenytoin and phenobarbitone. Phenytoin has been associated with vomiting, tremors and rashes in the breastfed baby. One case of methaemoglobinaemia has been reported in a baby whose mother was also taking phenobarbitone.

Tricyclic antidepressants According to one manufacturer, these are excreted in breast milk but are not metabolised in the young baby. This may theoretically result in accumulation. However, no side-effects in babies have been reported and it would seem safe for the breastfeeding mother to take these provided the dose is not too high and the baby continues to thrive.

Diuretics
Can decrease the milk supply. Otherwise no harmful effects have been reported.

Gastrointestinal drugs
Aloe Affected the bowels of twelve out of fourteen babies in one study.

Calomel Affected the bowels of seven out of fourteen babies in one study.

Cascara Affected the bowels of ten out of twenty-two babies in one study.

Danthron Said by the manufacturers to increase bowel activity in babies.

Phenolphthalein One study showed that the bowels of sixteen out of thirty-nine babies were affected, though two other studies showed no effect.

Senna Older senna preparations may affect a baby's bowels but Senokot appears to have no effect in usual doses.

Hormones and synthetic substitutes
Corticosteroids (steroids) Studies in humans so far are inadequate but

rat studies have shown death or growth retardation in sucklings after high daily doses. Most researchers advise against breast-feeding.

Corticotrophin Said to increase the potassium and decrease the sodium in breast milk.

Diethylstilboestrol If a 'dry-up' dose is given, the milk supply can easily be worked up again.

Oral contraceptives Oestrogen/progestogen combinations used in contraceptive doses can suppress lactation quite markedly. Two studies have shown a decrease in protein, fat and minerals in breast milk. Isolated reports exist of breast enlargement in male babies, proliferation of the vaginal epithelium in female babies and changes in bones, though these all occurred with higher dose oral contraceptives than are now used. One study, unconfirmed by others, showed a correlation between prior contraceptive use of these hormones and breast milk jaundice. Effects of the progestogen-only pill on babies who are breastfed are not fully known as yet, but the milk yield seems to be unaffected. It is too early as yet to be sure about the long-term safety with respect to cancer of oral contraceptives for the breastfed baby. Any drug is best avoided by the breastfeeding mother, so other forms of contraception (excluding hormone-containing intra-uterine contraceptive devices) must be preferable.

Miscellaneous drugs

Aspirin Large doses can cause rashes or gastrointestinal side-effects. It is thought to be safe for mothers of breastfed babies to take although it may be contra-indicated if the baby has a blood-clotting disorder.

Atropine Said to diminish milk flow and cause constipation and retention of urine in the baby but there is no good documentation of this.

Bismuth (in nipple cream) Should not be used.

Bromocriptine Suppresses lactation. The prolactin levels fall within a few hours.

Caffeine See page 126.

Digoxin Two recent reports conclude that even if the breastfeeding mother is on a high dose of digoxin the amounts secreted in breast milk are small and infant exposure is low.

Dihydrotachysterol Animal studies show decalcification of the bones. Some authors recommend that mothers taking this should not breastfeed.

Ergometrine Lowers prolactin levels. It has been suggested that multiple doses might suppress lactation. In some obstetric units ergometrine is now given after delivery only if the uterus fails to contract and to expel the placenta naturally (which often takes half an hour or so) or if there is post-partum bleeding from the uterus.

Ergot alkaloids 90 per cent of breastfed babies had signs of ergotism (diarrhoea and vomiting; weak pulse; unstable blood pressure) in one study. Many derivatives can suppress lactation.

Gold Can cause rashes and other 'odd' reactions.

Indomethacin One manufacturer recommends that this drug should not be given to breastfeeding mothers. There is one case report of convulsions in a breastfed baby whose mother took this drug.

Lead Lead toxicity (including encephalitis) has occurred after the use of lead acetate ointment on nipples and after the use of lead breast shields.

Mercury Mothers exposed to high levels should not breastfeed.

Nicotine May reduce the milk supply. There is one case report of restlessness and circulatory disturbance in a baby. Smoking breastfeeding mothers are more likely to give up breastfeeding early than non-smokers (see also page 126).

Phenylbutazone Use with caution because of the possibility of a blood dyscrasia.

Pyridoxine One study showed a decrease in the milk supply.

Propranolol Only small amounts appear in the milk of mothers taking this. However, because of the theoretical possibility of accumulation in the baby and because of the immaturity of the enzyme systems responsible for metabolism, close observation for heart slowing or low blood sugar is necessary.

Reserpine One report has been made of significant nasal stuffiness, slowing of the heart and some increase in tracheobronchial secretions.

Radioactive drugs

Experts differ in their advice to breastfeeding mothers but the following advice is a safe summary.

The following may be used for diagnostic testing or for treatment.

^{67}*Gallium citrate*[1] Significant amounts are excreted in milk. Different experts advise that breastfeeding should be interrupted for between 72 hours and two weeks.

^{125}*I labelled albumin*[2] Significant amounts are excreted. Avoid the drug or stop breastfeeding for at least ten days.

^{131}*I*[2] Breastfeeding should be interrupted for one to three weeks after a large therapeutic dose. After smaller, diagnostic doses, discard milk for at least twenty-four hours (or for seventy-two hours, according to one author).

^{131}*I labelled macroaggregated albumin*[2] Discard breast milk for ten to twelve days.

^{131}*I hippurate*[25] Discard breast milk for twenty-four hours.

^{99m}*TCO$_4$*[2] (technetium 99) Discard breast milk for 32 to 72 hours.

^{99m}*TCO$_4$ labelled macroaggregated albumin*[1] Discard breast milk for twenty-four hours.

If you are going to have any radioactive isotope investigation or treatment don't forget to tell the doctor that you're breastfeeding.

While breastfeeding is interrupted, keep your milk supply going by expressing or pumping milk frequently and discarding it. If the interruption is to be short, you can plan ahead and store expressed or pumped breast milk in the fridge or freezer to be given to the baby during that time. Sometimes tests involving radioactive materials can be avoided completely in the breastfeeding mother.

If you are taking any drug while breastfeeding, check with your doctor that it is not one of the above list. Of course, it's wisest always to remind your doctor that you are breastfeeding before he prescribes anything for you, as he may not know.

Radio-active fallout

There have been no proven cases of toxicity to breastfed babies from strontium 89 or 90 and caesium 137. Breast milk, in any case, has lower levels of these substances than does cows' milk.

Insecticides

DDT and PCBs (polychlorinated biphenyls) are thought to present no problem to the breastfed baby (although they can be present in breast milk) because the amounts involved are so small. In most cases, although insecticides can be present in breast milk, the levels are less than those in cows' milk and anyway have not exceeded safe limits. However, if there has been unusual exposure to such chemicals, the milk levels should be measured.

Hexachlorobenzene Many infant deaths occurred in Turkey after mothers ate wheat treated with this insecticide.

Immunisations

The 'triple' vaccine (diphtheria, pertussis/whooping cough, and tetanus) is not affected by breastfeeding and should be given to the breastfed baby at the normal recommended times. The same goes for polio, rubella, mumps, measles, yellow fever, cholera and typhoid vaccines.

Twins or more

Because two babies demand twice as much milk as one, you'll automatically make enough milk for them. Many mothers have breastfed twins successfully and happily for as long as they wanted to, so don't let anyone try to persuade you that you'll have to give either one or both of them cows' milk formula feeds.

To save time it's a good idea to get the knack of feeding them both at once, though there will be times when you'll enjoy the luxury of feeding them separately. There are several positions in which you can feed them together; for example, try holding each one with his legs under your arm in the football hold – cushions or pillows under their heads will take the weight off your arms. Make sure that you position them properly as your nipples may become sore if either baby is dragging on the breast. Once you get into the swing of feeding them both, you'll find it works well.

Should you alternate the breast that each twin feeds from? The usual advice is yes, so that the twin that sucks more strongly has the chance to stimulate each breast alternately. However, newborn animals usually choose 'their' nipple and stick to it, so it may be that human babies would prefer to do just that too. Certainly in the first few weeks of breastfeeding, if you always fed one baby from one breast and the other from the other, and if one baby sucked more strongly and so drank more milk each time, then you would find that your breasts were rather lopsided. Once the milk supply is established, the breasts almost always become more equal in size, so this difference is scarcely noticeable.

Should you wake the second baby for a feed every time the first baby wakes? The answer is 'yes' if you want to save time on feeds and 'no' if you would like the occasional chance to suckle one baby at a time. If you are at all unhappy about your milk supply then you should always wake the second baby and feed them both.

Many mothers have successfully breastfed triplets, though sometimes cows' milk formula is necessary as well, especially early on. However many babies you have, some breast milk is still good for them.

Re-starting your milk supply (relactation)
There are several reasons why you might want to do this. You may have decided initially not to breastfeed, only to change your mind after a few weeks. You may want to breastfeed an adopted baby. You may want to put your baby back on breast milk after an untimely weaning. In each case it's possible to build up your milk supply, though you'll need to persevere and also you'll need a cooperative baby!

If your baby has been on cows' milk formula for several weeks and your milk supply has dried up, the way to start it up again is by putting the baby to your breast frequently. He may become very frustrated at feeding from an empty breast, especially because the shape of the nipple is not such a strong stimulus to suck as the shape of a rubber teat. You can try two things. Either let him have some cows' milk formula from the bottle to allay his initial hunger pangs, then let him feed from you, or give him cows' milk formula from a spoon, so avoiding the stimulus of the rubber teat, then let him feed from you. When you have some milk back, try to get your let-down working before putting your baby to the breast. You may find a Lact-aid helpful (see below).

After each feed, express or pump your breasts to encourage the milk supply to build up. Remember that the more often the baby breastfeeds, the more quickly your milk will reappear. After about two weeks you will probably produce enough milk for him, so you can do away with cows' milk formula.

The keynote to success is confidence. Your breasts are quite capable of producing milk again even after several years of being dry, *as long as they have enough stimulation*.

A more unusual situation is if you want to breastfeed an adopted baby. Believe it or not, many women have fully breastfed adopted babies years after feeding their own babies, and some women have fed adopted babies without ever having been pregnant, though they needed to supplement their breast milk with other food.

Once your breasts have been prepared for lactation by a pregnancy they will always retain their ability to produce milk. If they have produced milk for any length of time, they'll be even more able to produce milk years later. This is why grandmothers in many parts of the world can breastfeed their grandchildren many years after feeding their own children.

Start building up your milk supply before the adopted baby arrives by expressing or pumping your breasts at frequent intervals. When the baby arrives, you'll probably need to give both cows' milk formula and your own milk unless he is lucky enough to have been breastfed until then by his mother. In this case you may be able to carry on giving him breast milk either from her, from a breast milk bank or from a breastfeeding friend until your milk becomes plentiful enough.

A useful piece of equipment for re-lactating mothers is the Lact-aid, which was developed by a man for his wife who successfully built up her milk supply to feed an adopted baby. This gadget delivers milk (breast milk or cows' milk formula) from a plastic bag (which you secure to your clothing) through a fine plastic tube which enters the baby's mouth with your nipple. Because the baby receives milk from the tube while feeding at your breast, he is happy and so continues feeding without getting frustrated. Your nipples also get the necessary stimulation to build up your milk supply. A useful instruction booklet is available from the distributor. (See page 267.)

How long will it take to build up your milk supply? It has been done within two weeks by mothers who weaned their own baby as long as six years before. It usually takes much longer. The pleasure it gives can far outweigh the difficulty involved, though you must be prepared for it to take some time.

14 Mainly for fathers

It's probably fair to say that many husbands don't care much whether their wives breastfeed or not. This is a pity because there are so many advantages for both mother and baby (as we've already seen) that most husbands would be hard pushed *not* to be convinced if they knew the whole story. But in addition to this there are positive advantages from their point of view.

While a baby gorilla is being born the father fusses about the mother and when she has given birth he lifts the baby up to her breast at once so that she can suckle it. As we've already seen, this would be difficult for most human fathers to do in the West because of the problems involved in hospital births. But it doesn't mean it's impossible. Once you and your wife have made the decision that she will breastfeed your baby and that you will encourage her, you should try to help right from the start.

We feel that even (or indeed especially) at this early stage you, the father, can take a positive hand in encouraging your baby to feed properly. Some hospitals give breastfed babies water, glucose water or cows' milk formula indiscriminately (especially at night) and you can help your wife prevent this from happening. The best thing to do is to tell the sister and the doctor that you both want your baby totally breastfed. You'll find it's best to tell them before the birth, preferably on admission to the maternity unit. A word of warning: don't be fobbed off. Midwives and doctors in some hospitals will try to persuade you that it doesn't matter if the baby has the odd bottle. However it's up to you to hold out for what *you* feel is right for *your* baby. Even one bottle of cows' milk formula can trigger off an allergic reaction either at the time or later in a susceptible child (usually with a family history of some kind of allergy), so it's well worth the effort.

If you do discuss this matter with the nursing or medical staff after the birth, make sure that you don't have any scenes in front of your wife as this could upset her and so make breastfeeding more difficult.

Having helped your wife get the baby to the breast, stay with her if at all possible. She's just been through the greatest event in her life and will want you as her partner and friend there for company and to share in the experience. We should like to see more hospitals giving a private half hour or more to parents with their new baby so they can share their pleasure before the pressures of everyday life impinge on them again.

It's right here in the delivery room that you start looking after your wife in a new way. She may not be able to take in everything that's going on if only because she's so emotionally and physically keyed up. It's an interesting fact that women who have difficult or unpleasant labours tend to be less likely to breastfeed, so everything you can do to help your wife, even this early on, will help her breastfeed more successfully. In the USA it's common practice to ask the woman if she'd like to breastfeed or not immediately after the birth and if the answer is 'no' then she is given an injection to dry up her milk there and then. (In some hospitals they aren't even asked, they simply get the injection!) Of course, most women are in no fit state to make a rational decision about a matter like this in the few minutes after giving birth and undoubtedly many women who would like to have fed their babies will have had their milk suppressed because they didn't want to say 'no' to anything the hospital suggested. This practice is not common in the UK where drugs are now only rarely used to dry up milk but there are parallels and the presence of a 'with it' father can be a great help. Even if the milk is dried up with drugs, she can still get her milk back if she changes her mind.

If your wife is going to have problems it's in the first week that they'll be worst. This is unfortunate because it's at this time that so many women feel at their lowest and need most help. One experienced breastfeeding counsellor has gone so far as to say that successful lactation depends on the woman's helpers and advisers and not on her ability to produce milk. Unfortunately some hospitals make new mothers feel bad by making them feel like a milk-producing appendage to the baby. Sometimes there is an internal conflict in the mind of the nurse or doctor who like to think of all the babies on the ward as 'theirs'. As soon as the mother shows any signs of having problems with feeding, they jump in with a bottle and so take over the baby. You should ensure that this doesn't happen.

But however useful you may be in the few days your wife may spend in hospital, your real help begins when she gets home. If you have other children you'll have been pretty busy looking after them already. Take a couple of weeks off work if you can, so that you can look after the other children and be around when your wife comes home.

Once home, your wife will need you as provider, protector and general helper. For breastfeeding to succeed you'll need to play a very important part in the life of the family for the next few weeks at least. This should be no hardship. After all, most of us have only two children in a lifetime so it should be no problem to give your wife the support and help she'll need during this crucial period.

Most women come home from hospital expecting to run the house exactly as before. Women tell us that they feel their poor husbands have already been coping with their other children long enough and need a rest themselves. If your wife is going to breastfeed successfully, don't be under any illusions: she'll need your help. Obviously you'll need to go on providing for her in a material sense but she'll also need a lot of love and emotional back-up.

Apart from providing a happy home environment you'll have to protect her from the children, from well-meaning but ill-informed busybodies and most of all from herself. Children will be no less demanding now than they were before the baby came and you'll need to keep them amused so that your wife can rest. It's a shame that some babies hardly get to know their mothers because there are so many other people making their own demands on her time. You must act as a buffer between her and the world around her. Relatives and neighbours will be keen to see the baby. Make sure they come in small doses. Many's the time a recently delivered mother gets so exhausted from regaling the world with her hospital sagas that she simply can't relate to or feed her new baby properly.

Breastfeeding is a deeply emotional business. Research studies the world over have shown that mammals of many species (and humans are no exception) simply produce less milk or even none at all if they are disturbed or stressed while breastfeeding. A woman has to become cow-like when feeding her baby, at least in the early weeks until lactation is really well established. Serenity is a must for really successful breastfeeding and it's up to you, her husband, to promote it.

Another thing you'll have to provide is encouragement. Studies have shown that women whose husbands don't want them to breastfeed rarely manage to do so. Even if the husband is merely 'neutral' the chances of successful feeding are greatly reduced. One American breastfeeding counsellor (who guarantees success) will not accept a woman as a client unless her husband approves of breastfeeding. So clearly it's best if you show a positive attitude right from the start. It can be more difficult to breastfeed than to bottle-feed in the first few days and your wife will need correspondingly more help which will throw new strains on to you.

To some degree the new father gets shut out of the excitement of the first few days. The new mother is so closely involved with her baby that he may well feel that the baby is hogging the limelight. Obviously this is true to some extent and it's only fair to let a woman revel in her new baby – but both mother and father have got to get used to a new person with all his physical and emotional demands and that's never easy. We're not suggesting for a moment that poor dad should become a pitiable figure that lurks in the shadows. On the contrary, although he'll have to do more than usual it is usually a wonderful time for both parents.

The majority of women are highly emotional after having a baby – their hormones keep them keyed up to respond to their babies. But as well as reacting to their baby's every whimper they may also react to the world around them in a way which is atypical for them. Even the toughest professional woman who has held down a big job may well collapse in tears for no apparent reason. Sometimes she'll do this because she's happy and this is very often difficult for a man to understand.

Just a little word of warning. Do be careful about what you say. Your wife will often be so dependent on you that almost anything you say might upset her. This is especially true when discussing breastfeeding. Husbands play a vital role in whether their wives carry on breastfeeding or not and often a casual, thoughtless remark can throw a woman completely and make her feel inadequate. Until breastfeeding is well and truly established be very sensitive about what you say!

Two of the things that worry husbands most about breastfeeding (or at least the two things they most often talk about, which isn't necessarily the same thing at all) are whether their wives will (a) go off sex and (b) lose their figures. The next chapter is all about sex and breastfeeding so more of that later but here let's look at the figure question. Whether most of the breastfeeding experts like it or not, men today think of breasts first and foremost as sexual objects. We get rather tired of the people who tell us that breasts are functional organs for feeding babies. Of course they are but not exclusively so and for the forty-odd years of the average couple's married life their erotic role is vastly more important. It seems ridiculous to pretend that husbands' fears about their wives having droopy breasts after feeding are unjustified.

All breasts enlarge during pregnancy regardless of whether the woman is going to breastfeed or not, but if she does feed her baby, her breasts will be bigger for longer. Strange as it may seem, the research into breast size after breastfeeding is scanty and confused. But overall one thing does emerge. Women who had breastfed for two weeks or more reported that their breasts had become slightly droopier. They also felt that overall the pleasure they had from feeding their babies far outweighed this change in their figure. Had they known the medical arguments for breastfeeding they would without a doubt have been even less concerned about the long-term effects on their breasts than they were.

But does this change really matter? Did you, you should ask yourself, marry your wife simply for her breasts? And how many women that you see walking around who've had children have such unattractive breasts that you don't want to look at them? The quest for 'perfect' breasts is not only a little crazy but it's also thoroughly unrealistic because most of us don't marry girls out of the centre spread of *Playboy* in the first place. Breasts quite naturally change with age and breastfeeding might just hasten this change a little, if at all.

A lot of fathers tell us that they like the idea of their wives breastfeeding but feel it leaves them with little they can do for the baby. If that's the case it's a shame because having a baby is a joint affair and enjoying it should be too. Whether you give the baby the odd feed or two is really beside the point. Any father who thinks he'll get nothing positive out of his child being breastfed should think again because there are lots of ways in which he'll benefit.

First, he'll never have to get up at night to prepare a feed and that's no mean advantage when he's at work again. The family can't run out of milk powder at awkward times either. Breastfeeding does make extra demands on the mother's body and so she has to eat more than normal, but even allowing for the cost of these extra calories breastfeeding is still less expensive than formula feeding according to three major studies. But whatever artificial milk costs it's one thing less you'll have to remember to buy and means there are fewer baby things to carry when you go out anywhere.

Last of all and probably most important is the pleasure it'll give you. You'll get this by seeing your wife happy, content and fulfilled by being a real 'female' mother. Many women revel in this feeling of femininity and their husbands often benefit from it too.

But there are still many husbands who feel they won't have as much fun with and won't be as close to their new baby as they would have been if they had been helping with the bottle feeding. This is a sad argument because there are lots of other things a father can do: he can cuddle his baby, play with him, bath and change him for instance.

You may feel that we've made it all sound rather hard going for the new breastfeeding dad! If we have, it's only to point out some of the ways in which you can help your wife do something that'll bring pleasure to you both and give your baby the best start he could get in life. Just think of all the time and money you're going to lavish on your children over the years yet so many husbands seem to cheesepare their time and affection in the first vital weeks. If you do help your wife, it'll really make a big difference.

15 Breastfeeding and sex

In all the books, learned medical papers and popular magazine articles that have been written about breastfeeding, few until recently said much (if anything) about breastfeeding as a sexual experience. Yet the deep-seated sexual nature of breastfeeding is only too apparent to many women. The trouble is that we live in a repressed society even in this so-called permissive age and many women feel guilty linking any sexual pleasure they may feel with breastfeeding. If they experience anything more than a pleasant feeling they are uneasy and often intensely guilty because 'everyone knows that no one but your husband should arouse feelings like that'. It's because this guilt and other sexual hang-ups are such common causes for the failure of breastfeeding that we've devoted a whole chapter to the subject.

When you think about it, breastfeeding, like intercourse, must have been pleasurable throughout history or the human species would never have kept going as successfully as it has! If there are two things that had to be pleasant to ensure humanity's continuance, sex and breastfeeding were they.

The link between sexual pleasure and breastfeeding comes as a bolt from the blue to many women and even positively revolts some. A psychosexual specialist with knowledge of this subject once made a television broadcast in which he suggested that some women actually had an orgasm when breastfeeding – a well-documented occurrence although by no means a common one. The switchboard was jammed with outraged women, one of whom phoned to say she had actually vomited while he was talking. It's this sort of attitude, though usually repressed, that makes a lot of women either not breastfeed at all or fail when they do. Feelings of sexuality are acceptable to most of us only within certain very strict bounds; and breastfeeding a baby comes outside them!

To see why this is contrary to what nature intended and why such cultural taboos hinder breastfeeding, let's look at some basic and undeniable facts. To a man, sex means intercourse. If he is making love to a woman he loves and who is the mother of his children, so much the better. But often men say how readily they can enjoy intercourse with a woman who means little or nothing to them. Men are relatively simple in their sexual demands and relatively easily pleased.

To a woman, on the other hand, sex means much more. True, some women are like men and can centre their sex lives on their genitals but this is uncommon. To most women sexuality is much more complex and enduring and often a more emotional business than it is for a man. A woman's sexuality starts to blossom in her teens and soon she is on her way to looking for a loving, considerate sex partner and possibly a father for her potential children. Her sexuality takes an even more fulfilling and dramatic turn when she becomes pregnant and carries a baby around inside her for several months. Her body changes in numerous ways, as does her mind, and many experts say that she never feels the same again: she's felt something she's never experienced before, and her relationship with her child gives her a new outlook on life and herself.

At the end of pregnancy she gives birth to a baby – another remarkable physical and emotional experience – and then feeds it. Or does she?

Primitive women were ruled by their cycles. Breastfeeding did, and still does, perform a more important role as a contraceptive than all the man-made methods put together; indeed, this is how families are spaced by most solely breastfeeding peoples. Many millions of women the world over are either pregnant or lactating for the whole of their reproductive lives and are ruled by their hormones from when their periods start until the menopause.

Today's western woman doesn't want to be ruled by her hormones and social changes have made her loath to have babies every two or three years, spaced only by breastfeeding contraception. Today's woman wants to be free to behave more like a man and society does everything possible to ensure that this happens. This move started in earnest in the 1920s when women began to become an important economic force in the developed countries. Union leaders, industrialists and parents today all agree that life is becoming so expensive in the western world that it is scarcely possible for one breadwinner per family to cope. Indeed, many industries now depend on female labour: the UK would probably grind to a halt if women were not in the work force. More than half of all the married women in the UK work at least part-time.

Women have therefore come to expect more education, to work for at least a part of their lives, to put off getting married and having children and generally to try – often against their will, it's true – to behave more like men. And we're not just talking about feminists. This attitude is now common in almost every stratum of society.

All right, we can hear you say. That's all very well but women are equal to men and so deserve equal opportunity. True. But one way in which they're very *different* from men is in their hormones. Modern society has tried to make women the same as men when their whole physiological make-up is different, and whether we like it or not we are still ruled by the basic laws of nature. If we ignore these laws we must expect to pay the price. It's partly because modern women are by and large loath to be *female* any more (although they are probably more *feminine* than ever) that breast-feeding has declined in popularity. Breastfeeding makes a woman realise that she really is a *woman* and that isn't very fashionable today as we've just seen.

Once we understand how a woman's whole make-up revolves around her hormones we're in a much better position to understand how to make breastfeeding successful in today's society and also to see how closely it's linked with sex.

Although most people don't realise it, there's a tremendous similarity between a woman's periods, pregnancies, orgasms and lactation. During all of these her breasts become bigger, for a start. Most women also feel protective or 'motherly' after intercourse, after giving birth and during breastfeeding. This is no accident and stems from the fact that a woman's sex hormones act on several parts of her body at once and in different situations. For instance, oxytocin, the hormone that we've seen to be so crucial for the let-down reflex, is also released during orgasm and at birth.

However much we choose to deny it, a woman's sexuality is often linked to a feeling of motherliness. Today, though, it's fashionable to stress only the mechanics of sex and, as a result, magazine articles abound with hints on achieving the perfect orgasm and attaining niney-five different love positions. This quest for perfect orgasms (and preferably plenty of them) is an unconscious substitute for many of the other *female* joys that so many women now get either not at all, or very late in life (in biological terms).

Today, a woman's breasts have taken on a far more important role in the eyes of most people: a sexual one. Breasts have become the erotic focus for most western men and are now an integral part of the fabric of modern society. When did you last see a foot advertising a new cigar? No one knows why certain societies home in on a particular part of the female anatomy in this way but it's interesting that we are the only mammal in which the female's breasts develop before they're actually needed to feed the young. There's no reason to suppose, though, that it's because of this that they have taken on an erotic role; in fact, we in the West are unusual among our fellow men in placing such erotic value on the breast.

So, with men putting such a sexual emphasis on the breast, is it surprising that sexual overtones often militate very strongly against breastfeeding? Studies show that many women won't even consider breastfeeding simply because they believe it will ruin their breasts and so make them less sexually attractive. If you find this difficult to believe, bear in mind that just about the commonest subject on which agony columnists in the women's press receive letters is that of breast size and you'll soon see that there really is a problem.

Many women get sexual pleasure from breast stimulation by their partners or themselves and studies show that some women can actually experience an orgasm from breast stimulation alone. This is scarcely surprising as the clitoris, uterus and nipples are interconnected by nerves via the brain. So not only do women's hormones (mostly oxytocin) link these organs but her nervous pathways do too.

Let's look first at the sexual feelings a woman gets when breastfeeding. For women who relate easily to their bodies, breastfeeding is often a pleasurable experience. For them, at worst it's a pleasant, relaxing way of feeding a baby but at best it's sometimes a stimulating event which 'turns them on'. All shades in between are completely normal and, as one would expect, most women will fall somewhere between the two. Replies to those who ask the right questions show that many breastfeeding women feel sexually aroused albeit in a controlled and simple way. Some notice some vaginal lubrication and a few actually have an orgasm. We get the impression that breastfeeding engenders more positively enjoyable feelings in women than they admit to, even to themselves. Whilst most women certainly do not have an orgasm while breastfeeding, many describe a parallel experience which is less explosive and more calming. They also get a feeling of euphoria or well-being after a feed which is much like that after an orgasm.

Some women say that they find breastfeeding so sexually pleasing that they feel more sexy towards their husbands. In fact, it's well known that breastfeeding women return to sexual intercourse sooner after birth than do their bottle-feeding sisters. Certainly the breastfeeding woman returns to normal physically more quickly but it's also likely that the repeated feelings of sexual arousal (however minimal they are) also make her more receptive to sex. Some studies show that a substantial number of women are more sexually active when breastfeeding than at any other time. This is good news for fathers who may feel left out at this time!

However, even if a woman gets pleasure from having her baby at her breast, her husband may not enjoy the baby's relationship with his wife. Until now he hasn't had to share his wife's breasts and he may resent the little intruder. As we've already mentioned, a husband can actually put a woman off feeding successfully simply by being negative, but he shouldn't be blamed. So many things make him think of her breasts as erotic that it's hardly surprising that he'll feel bad about somebody usurping his place, especially since that somebody is now taking up most of her time and love.

The thing is to be positive. Show your husband you still love and want him. Don't let him feel that, because the baby's feeding, that's all you see your breasts as doing. Let your husband play with your breasts as he did before. He can even drink your milk if he wants to: he won't be robbing the baby of anything. Should you feel sexually aroused by breastfeeding, this can be pleasant for your partner too. This brings us to the negative side of the whole story because these pleasant feelings make some women feel guilty.

Most women are shy of their breasts. Strange though it may seem in an age where breasts assault us from all sides, women are very insecure about them. Men look at beautiful girls because they get a simple animal pleasure from them; women look at them to see what other women have that they haven't. And usually it's breasts they're comparing. If society encouraged topless bathing, naturist beaches and open display of the breast in fashion, then perhaps women would not feel so shy but the fact is, they still do. It's this feeling of shyness, propriety and frank prudery that puts many women off starting to breastfeed.

But even if most women could overcome this aversion to showing their breasts, a substantial proportion simply don't like their breasts touched or played with even by their partners, let alone by a champing baby. Dr Kinsey found that up to 50 per cent of all non-pregnant women found breast stimulation unpleasant or sexually unarousing. In such cases there's precious little a book like this can do. Indeed, we know some women who are completely revolted by the whole idea of suckling a baby at all and it's nearly impossible to convince them that it will be *pleasant*. Only another woman who once felt the same way but later changed her mind can do that.

Breastfeeding succeeds best in 'breast-orientated' *female* women who like their breasts and like having them touched. A study in the USA found that women who failed to breastfeed had substantially more sexual hang-ups than those who succeeded. Another piece of research showed that 65 per cent of women who successfully breastfed 'positively enjoyed the experience', but that still left 35 per cent who didn't. Most of these found it unpleasant because they thought it 'immodest' and 'distasteful'.

For most women, the comparison with cows doesn't go unnoticed and in today's so-called sophisticated society this can be a considerable turn-off. It really isn't an unreasonable comparison, though, because lactating women *are* like cows if they are lactating cows! So what, though? Cows also walk around in fields yet that doesn't stop us going for country walks.

Some women feel less sexy when breastfeeding. The inevitable tiredness that comes with waking at night means that many a breastfeeding woman falls asleep as soon as her head hits the pillow. To her, sleep is more important than sex. Making love in the morning after waking up will be impossible if the baby or other young children are awake too, so the couple may find themselves having intercourse infrequently. Breast tenderness (especially a long time after a feed) can make breast play painful and this can turn them off sex. One possible way round this is to breastfeed before intercourse. Some women point out that their nipples don't erect as much as they used to and that they lose sexual pleasure because of this. This is in fact an illusion. The nipples do erect in a lactating woman but their increase in size can be masked by the already swollen breast. It's the same with breast size. Some women get pleasure from the swelling of their breasts when they're stimulated during sex play. The lactating breast doesn't swell as much (because it's already so big) and this can make the woman feel that she's not responding in the usual way.

A few women find their relationship with their baby so physically and emotionally satisfying that they simply don't need physical contact and emotional support from their husband. They should realise what is happening and try to understand how their husbands must feel about this, especially in our monogamous society!

Some couples find that the women's breasts get in the way or are painful in certain lovemaking positions. This can easily be overcome by changing to another position and anyway is a problem only for about the first two months. Another problem is that during intense sexual excitement milk may spurt or leak from your nipples. This can be exciting for the man but some people don't like it simply because it can be so messy. If this upsets you or your partner, try feeding the baby before you make love to reduce the likelihood of spurting.

The foundation stones of successful breastfeeding are laid early on in a couple's married life and even probably during courtship. Whilst it's by no means a common subject of honeymoon conversation, the more a man plays with his wife's breasts, stimulates them and makes sure she likes it, the better the chances that she will even consider breastfeeding when the time comes. Remember, the size and shape of your breasts and nipples have no bearing on the enjoyment you and your husband will get from them – and this goes for the baby too.

During pregnancy we suggest that the only nipple care that should take place at all for normal nipples is that carried out by your husband. Get him to roll them gently between his fingers or in his mouth during love play.

Breastfeeding itself shouldn't interfere with sexual intercourse – and it had better not because you may be breastfeeding for several months and probably much longer if you want to. Any husband who gives the ultimatum 'baby or me' is doing all three of you a great disfavour. If you really feel strongly about feeding your baby even though it's at a very late stage, try to persuade your husband. Tell your husband that he and the baby will be able to share your breasts.

Childbirth, especially the birth of the first child, is a big upheaval for your husband. If anything, it's easier for you because you've got all the joys (and work!) of looking after the baby. Your husband is often only an interested bystander. Here are a few hints on how to combine a good sex life with a happy breastfeeding baby.

1 Make sure your husband doesn't feel left out, physically or emotionally. You've got the baby to cuddle; who has he got?
2 If feeding makes you feel sexy or even just pleasantly relaxed, tell him so to encourage him to make the most of it.
3 If you wear a bra at night tell him you're doing it so that your breasts will look good years from now. Take it off to make love.
4 Respect his wishes not to feed in public or in front of certain people if you know it upsets him.
5 Plan the odd trip out together as soon as you feel happy taking the baby around and feeding in public places or in front of strangers. You can't expect your husband to look favourably on breastfeeding if he thinks he's going to be tied to the house for the next six months.
6 Keep up your previous 'mistress' image as much as possible.
7 Talk to one another about how you feel breastfeeding is affecting your relationship, for good or bad.

Whether or not a woman is likely to choose to breastfeed (let alone continue to do so, once started) depends very greatly upon the psychosexual make-up of her partner. In research we have done among 300 women of all ages we have found that the majority (about three quarters) were dissatisfied with their breasts. Obviously, a woman who feels negatively about her breasts is less likely to see them as suitable or worthy things for her baby. Just why so many women feel this way about their breasts isn't known but the trouble undoubtedly starts in teenage life as the girl's body image is beginning to grow. Because of society's rather stereotyped attitude to breasts many women feel they can't match up to the mythical 'ideal' breast of the girlie magazines and advertising photos and so begin to feel negatively towards their own. Men may unthinkingly hasten this downhill process but our research shows that a man will usually be much more satisfied with his partner's breasts than she thinks he is.

Another psychosexual problem with breastfeeding is that many men imagine their wife to have only a fixed store of love and affection – a store which will have to be shared one more way when she's breastfeeding a new baby. What they need is someone to tell them that this doesn't necessarily mean that they'll get a smaller slice of the 'love cake'! The cake can actually grow so that the old slice stays the same (in spite of another slice coming out) or even grow. Many couples have told us how common this is.

Unfortunately, there are other psychosexual problems. In the western world, partly because of the Christian Church's influence over the centuries, men have come to have two images of their women – images that are often mutually exclusive, except in a very psychosexually balanced and mature person. These images are of the madonna and the mistress.

When a couple meet and get married the man sees his partner as a mistress, which indeed she is. When children come along she becomes the madonna – an untouchable, sexless, slightly revered person on a pedestal with her baby. Breastfeeding of course reinforces the madonna image because that's what madonnas do.

Many men, then, lose their mistress when she starts having babies, yet don't much want to gain a madonna. In a monogamous society this can lead to all kinds of sexual and interpersonal stress in a marriage and by breastfeeding (especially for a long time) the woman is seen in the eyes of such men to be almost flaunting her madonna image – to his detriment.

This situation can also present problems for women, some of whom have adapted to the mistress role and now find themselves in a rather different one. A woman after childbirth may want 'mothering' by her husband (as her mother is so often not there) but he won't feel like being a mother, especially as he has just lost a mistress.

All of this is very complex and in today's society is often a potent factor in the failure to start or to continue breastfeeding. When a man says, 'I think you've fed the baby long enough', or 'When are you going to get back to normal?', he means, 'When are you going to be my mistress again?' As the couple mature together such problems tend to diminish. Could this be why so many women fail to feed a first baby yet do so successfully with later-borns?

All of these problems can be reduced, if not totally demolished, by frank discussion between the couple and by realising that many others feel exactly the same. Some will need professional help to sort things out. It makes sense for a woman to retain as much of her mistress image as possible when breastfeeding, especially if her husband was hooked on that image beforehand. There really is no need to force a man to choose between you as madonna or mistress, except maybe for a very short time either side of the baby's birth. And any loving man should be able to cope with that twice in a lifetime.

16 Feeding the older baby

Weaning

The verb 'to wean' comes from a word meaning 'to accustom'.
Many people think of 'weaning' only as taking a baby off breast milk
as other foods and drinks are introduced. However, we also like to
think of it as getting a baby used to (i.e. accustoming him to) other
foods while he is still being breastfed. Just because you start giving
your baby tastes of your family food doesn't mean to say that you
have to start weaning him from the breast. When, how and why you
wean are entirely up to you, though we think it's important to
discuss some important points, including the foods you give your
baby to replace your breast milk.

When should you wean?

Take no notice of the various pamphlets and baby books you read
which give you precise instructions as to the exact age or weight
your baby should be when you start weaning. There is no such age
or weight and there are no hard and fast rules.

As long as your baby is thriving, happy and gaining weight
regularly and as long as you are both enjoying it, carry on breastfeeding him.

It's easier to say when you shouldn't start weaning! Breast milk
alone is the best food for your baby for at least the first three months
and for longer if he is satisfied. If you introduce cows' milk formula
and solids before three months you are not only laying yourself open
to the possibility of reducing your milk supply, but you are also
laying your baby open to the chance of foreign protein leaking into
his bloodstream via his gut lining and possibly causing sensitisation
if he is susceptible. This, as we've seen, may lead to the development of allergies.

There are two ways of introducing other foods: either you can wait until your baby shows a real interest in the food the rest of the family is eating and let him pick up some of this food with his fingers, or you can give him spoonfuls of food. The first way would seem to be the most sensible, though if left to themselves some babies might carry on with breast milk alone for rather longer than would seem nutritionally advisable. Some breastfed babies thrive on breast milk alone for eight months or even more.

If it's left to the baby to decide when he wants to start finger feeding, he'll probably try at about six months or so. As this is also the age at which many babies get their first tooth, it seems likely that this is roughly the age nature intended babies to start on foods other than breast milk.

There's no need to offer him spoonfuls of food before six to eight months if he's thriving, as breast milk will provide adequate amounts of nutrients for the majority of babies till then. Later in the second half of the first year your baby will need more than breast milk alone can provide, though there is no need to give large amounts of food straight away; increase it slowly as he wants it.

One exception to this general rule is the premature baby whose liver stores of iron may not be large enough to last for six months until other foods are introduced. Iron is stored in the baby's liver in the last few weeks of pregnancy in particular, so if the baby is born early he may not have enough iron to last for six months on milk alone. It's an easy enough matter for your doctor to test a drop of your baby's blood to see if there is any danger of anaemia developing.

Iron supplements can be given if necessary, though in practice they rarely are necessary for the fully breastfed baby. It's a fact that premature bottle-fed babies are more likely to become anaemic than premature breastfed babies, even though the level of iron in modified cows' milk is higher than that in breast milk. This is because breast milk iron is better absorbed than cows' milk iron.

Once you have introduced other foods, you can carry on breast-feeding as long as your baby wants and as long as your milk supply lasts. Some mothers find their babies lose interest in the breast relatively soon while others find their babies don't seem to want to give it up at all. The milk supply should last as long as you want it to if you are giving your baby much of his fluid in this way. If you give him lots of other drinks and only one or two breastfeeds a day, your milk will slowly dry up, though some mothers give only a single feed for many months and find it's a sure way of helping their babies settle down at night.

There is no hard-and-fast rule of how long lactation will last. As long as the baby is stimulating your breasts, they'll produce some milk. Wet nurses used to carry on feeding for years on end and many mothers the world over feed their children for several years. The western idea that milk automatically dries up after a few months is totally wrong: 70 per cent of the world's population breastfeed for more than nine months and the average time a baby is breastfed in developing countries is two to three years.

What are the advantages of carrying on breastfeeding after six months? First, your baby will continue to receive protection against infection though full breastfeeding gives this advantage only for eight months, after which time, from the infection point of view, your baby is just as well off without your milk. In fact, babies fully breastfed (with no additional food) for longer than eight months are at greater risk from infection than babies who are being weaned by then, so this is one argument for introducing solids by eight months.

Second, you and your baby probably enjoy feed times together and will be extremely disappointed to give them up. Breastfeeding offers your baby emotional as well as nutritional sustenance; an older baby often turns to the breast to find comfort when he is upset. Many mothers remember their very real feelings of loss when they gave their baby his last breastfeed and they also remember their anguish and the tears and frustration of the baby denied the breast because it was felt to be the 'right' time to wean. There is no need for anguish on either your part or your baby's. *Simply let him decide when he wants to stop feeding and go along with him.* This is what is known as '*baby-led*' weaning. Whether he gives up the breast at nine months or eighteen, or even later, by doing it when he's ready he'll be happier than if you make him give it up.

So the answer to the question when to wean is not as simple as you might have thought. Solids should be introduced not earlier than three months and ideally not later than eight months but breastfeeding can continue for as long as you and your baby both want it to.

How to stop breastfeeding

If you have to stop breastfeeding for some reason, it's far easier if you do it gradually, almost without thinking about it. If you try to stop quickly, you'll probably end up with a fractious baby and painful, engorged breasts. There is no place for drying-up pills today – they have certain unpleasant side-effects and are unnecessary anyway.

Give up the feed at which you have least milk first. This is usually one in the later afternoon or early evening. Give your baby something else to drink instead: some mothers have strong feelings against bottles and get their babies drinking from a cup as soon as they start weaning. If you have to wean early, it's worth remembering that babies enjoy sucking and a bottle may be more enjoyable for him than a cup. If you're weaning later and intend letting your baby breastfeed when he wants to for comfort, if not for milk, then give him a drink from a cup.

After a week or so, give up another feed and and carry on in this way until you are feeding only once a day. You may find that it is most comfortable to give up the early morning feed last, as you'll probably have most milk at this feed. Some mothers like to give up the last feed of the day last of all, as their babies seem to enjoy this the most and sleep well afterwards.

Weaning should be unhurried and unworried. Certainly if you can possibly avoid it, don't ever wean in an emergency – there is almost always a way round the problem. Your baby would find it very hard to understand why he was suddenly denied the breast and might be upset for some time.

If your baby asks for a feed by nuzzling against your breast several days after you have stopped feeding him, let him feed. He'll soon realise that there is little, if any, milk there, though he may want to suck for comfort if not for food.

Don't forget that if you feel you've stopped breastfeeding too early, you can always get your milk supply back.

What should your baby eat?

If your baby's first foods are 'finger foods', foods that he can pick up himself with his hands and suck on or bite, then the choice of food is great. Let him have any raw fruit such as a large piece of peeled apple or banana, a rusk of baked wholemeal bread, or anything hard that won't be likely to break into pieces and choke him. He'll eat it by gradually dissolving it in his mouth.

If you're starting off with spoonfuls of food, remember that at first he won't be able to chew anything, so the food must be soft enough to swallow.

Whatever the method of feeding, the basic principles behind a healthy diet for your baby are the same. He'll do best on a varied diet containing protein, fat, carbohydrate, minerals and vitamins. At first he'll still be getting most of his food from your milk, so you needn't worry about giving him a balance of these nutrients until breast milk plays a less important role in his diet.

Some important points to realise are that it is quite unnecessary for a baby (or indeed anyone) to eat any added sugar. Sugar can rot the teeth, cause rapid swings in blood sugar and make people fat without contributing anything worthwhile or irreplaceable to the diet. Natural sugar in fruit and vegetables will taste quite sweet enough to your baby and if you can help him grow up without a sweet tooth you'll be doing him a great favour. Similarly, it's far better to give your baby unrefined carbohydrates: there is no need for him to have white, refined flour in any form, be it in cakes, biscuits, bread, puddings or rusks. Cook with wholemeal flour and you'll be standing him in good stead for the future. A diet high in unrefined carbohydrates will help protect a person from bowel and other disease for the rest of his life. A baby brought up on a diet which contains unrefined carbohydrate (rich in dietary fibre) and very little sugar will also be unlikely to get fat, which is another plus point.

Another thing best avoided is salt. Salt can actually be dangerous for a young baby if given in excess. It's worth remembering that your older baby will enjoy his food just as much without salt added and he will lose nothing by not having it.

Today's consumer society buys vast amounts of packaged, processed foods which bear little resemblance to their natural state.

Colourings, flavourings, emulsifiers, stabilisers, bleaches and many other chemicals are added to these foods and the public buys them with delight as many are so easy to prepare and look so bright and cheerful. Ideally, it would be better if you only gave your baby natural foods, without any commercial interference in the form of food additives. Although there is legislation regulating the use of these chemicals, many legal additives have recently come under the suspicion of being harmful. What is more, some are banned in some countries but not in others. Much more research is necessary before certain additives can be pronounced truly safe, so you and your family are better off avoiding them.

There's no need to use tinned or dried baby foods. Simply give your baby whatever you are going to eat, mashed or sieved first.

If you live in an area with low levels of fluoride in the drinking water, you may want to give the baby fluoride supplements in the form of tablets or drops. Ask your dentist about the local water and the amount of fluoride you should be giving. Fluoride cuts tooth decay by half.

One question frequently asked is whether a baby needs cows' milk once he's weaned from the breast. The answer is no. There is nothing in cows' milk which he can't get from other food sources provided he has a balanced diet. Even if he had no cheese or butter he would still be all right. If he likes milk, though, let him drink it.

As many of us live in a relatively sunless climate, some doctors advise giving pre-school children extra vitamin D as a daily supplement. Vitamin D is normally formed in the skin by the action of sunlight but it is possible to become deficient if shut indoors all day. Vitamin C is often included with vitamin D supplements which is just as well because so many people destroy dietary vitamin C by cooking their food too long. Be careful to give only the recommended amounts of vitamin D as it's harmful to give too much.

What drinks should your baby have to replace your milk? As we've said, he doesn't have to have cows' milk. The most popular drink for young children seems to be orange squash or blackcurrant syrup diluted with water. These syrups or squashes contain a lot of sugar, often with other additives such as colourings and flavourings, and are highly likely to cause tooth decay. While some of these drinks do contain vitamin C (one of the reasons mothers have for giving them) not all do and many contain no natural fruit juice at all. Your baby will do very well if you give him only water to drink. If you want to give something else for a change, give him the juice of an orange diluted with water or on its own. Apple juice is also popular.

Breastfeeding the older child

In this country the vast majority of breastfed babies are weaned from the breast by a year but there is no reason why you should do this if you don't want to. An increasing number of mothers are breastfeeding for longer periods – some until their children are two, three or even older.

Breastfeeding the older child is more important for the psychological comfort and pleasure it gives than for the nutritional value which is by then supplied in most cases in the western world at least by other foods. There is often little pattern to the feeds: the child comes for a drink when he feels like cuddling and being close to his mother, perhaps when he is upset or tired.

You may notice a difficult patch between four and six months when you wonder whether you really want to go on feeding. You'll feel this way for several reasons. First, you're feeling so much livelier in yourself that you want to get going again in the outside world; second, your baby will be more demanding and more aware and may cry more; third, he may be demanding more to eat and so make you feel you haven't got enough milk. Lastly, you may feel that breastfeeding is going to go on for ever and so may become disenchanted with it.

Don't get dispirited. If you really feel you've had enough of breastfeeding, give up gradually as we've suggested. It's better that you stop and carry on developing a loving relationship with your baby than start to resent feeding him.

If you continue breastfeeding as your baby passes the year stage, your only problem will be coping with uncalled-for criticism from friends, neighbours and relatives. Many of them will be surprised that you actually want to go on doing it for so long after other mothers have stopped! This can be very off-putting but if you and your baby want to go on, it's really none of their business.

To spare their amazement and your embarrassment, you may

ind it a good idea to feed your older baby alone. It's scarcely
surprising that a society which finds it hard to cope with the sight of
a little baby being breastfed finds it even more difficult to cope with
an older breastfed child. If your child tugs at your clothes or asks for
a feed when you are out visiting, if this is what you would prefer go
into another room to feed him. Don't make him feel there is
anything shameful in what you are doing and don't feel ashamed
yourself either!

However long you feed your baby you'll know you've done the
best thing for him and will almost certainly have enjoyed it yourself.
Just how long you go on for is very much a matter of personal choice
- there are no rules and no known physical benefits in the west after
about eight months. Don't let this put you off going on being a good
mother and whatever the experts say and however many fads come
and go, good mothering will always be at the heart of happy family
life.

Can you breastfeed while you are having a period?

The answer is 'yes'. There is no reason why you shouldn't as it won't
harm you or the baby. Some mothers say that their babies are rather
fractious around period time. This is quite likely to be due to their
own pre-menstrual tension being communicated to their babies,
rather than to any difference in the milk. Some babies have
diarrhoea for a couple of days, though, and others temporarily
reject the breast.

Changes in milk volume may occur during a period because of the
alteration in the blood flow through the breasts.

Can you breastfeed if you are pregnant?

You can breastfeed right through a pregnancy if you want to.

A few pregnant mothers experience pain in their breasts or
nipples, while others have feelings of aversion to their older baby or
child.

Some mothers find that their breast milk tends to diminish
during pregnancy. This is probably because the circulating pregnancy hormones affect milk production. The milk changes in
quality to become richer in fats and vitamins, so it is in no way
inferior even though its volume may be less. A month before the end

of pregnancy your milk supply will automatically increase.

A mother can carry on feeding her toddler along with the new baby. This can present problems if the toddler is allowed first call on the breast, as the baby may not get enough to drink, especially if the mother herself is undernourished. In some developing countries, weaning the older child is hazardous as there is often not enough food for the family and the toddler might easily become undernourished without his breast milk.

Breastfeeding two children of different ages at once is known as tandem nursing. Tandem nursing is a way of avoiding abrupt or untimely (from the baby's point of view) weaning of an older baby if another baby comes along while he is still being breastfed.

The way to manage natural breastfeeding is to do away with any rules and regulations and to be led as far as possible by your own baby and by your common sense. Let breastfeeding your baby be followed by baby-led weaning if you possibly can – you'll both find it easier.

17 Some common questions and answers

Q   Is it really necessary to eat more while breastfeeding?

A   Yes, it is. If you eat an extra 300 to 500 calories daily this still means that you're drawing on your own fat supplies to feed your baby. So if you are fairly slim anyway, you will need to eat even more than this. In fact, the Department of Health in the UK currently recommends an extra 600 calories a day while breast-feeding.

One survey found that stopping breastfeeding because of 'not enough milk' was less likely in a group of mothers who had been actively encouraged to eat more compared with a group who had had no such advice. Not all breastfeeding mothers feel a need for extra food, though it's interesting that those who breastfeed for longer tend to have larger appetites compared with their normal ones.

Q   I am pregnant and breastfeeding my first child, who is still taking quite a lot of milk from me. Will my next baby be deprived of the special benefits of colostrum when he is born because I am already producing mature milk?

A   No one knows whether the large volumes of milk you are already making will be enriched by the extra antibodies, protein, zinc and other minerals, vitamins A, E, B_6 and B_{12} and live cells found in colostrum. However, this research is being started now. It seems highly unlikely that your baby would be at any disadvantage and certainly even mature breast milk would be better for him than cows' milk formula.

Q   My baby spends a large amount of time during a feed just holding the nipple in his mouth without sucking. Is this normal?

A   Yes. It's partly caused by your let-down pattern (see page 15) but one researcher has also noted that 'newborn infants write their signature with their sucking rhythm, showing a constant, individual pattern in the number of sucks and intervals between sucks per minute'. This also helps explain why some babies take longer over a feed than others.

In general, 'nutritive' sucking is slower and stronger than 'non-nutritive' sucking. However, non-nutritive sucking (during which the baby swallows very little) is important both for the stimulation of milk production, the stimulation of a further let-down of milk in the feed, and for the comfort of the baby.

Q I've tried everything but my baby still cries in the early evening and isn't satisfied at the breast. Otherwise he is quite happy and gaining weight well. Is there anything I can do?
A It's been suggested by some experts that the milk supply may fall in the late afternoon and early evening if you don't have anything to eat between lunch time and supper time. Many women give their babies several feeds without thinking of feeding themselves to 'make the milk'. Try making it a habit to have something nutritious to eat between each of your baby's feeds.

Don't forget that old stand-by – a sling to carry your baby in while you are getting on with other things. A sling is useful in the home as well as when you're out. Your movements together with your body's warmth, sounds and closeness may make your baby more content. You can talk or sing to him as well. The one thing that never seems to work at this time of the day is putting the baby down in his cot and expecting him to amuse himself or go to sleep. Many experienced mothers expect to carry their babies around or sit and cuddle them for several hours at some time during the day. Young babies like to be with their mothers and if they're feeling irritable then it's especially no time to push them away. Of course, if you have extra pairs of hands around, then things are easier. Either that person can help with your other tasks or, if the baby is content, they can hold or play with him. This is why mothers who have a baby and one or more children old enough to be a help find looking after the baby so much easier. If your husband or another adult is around and willing to help, better still.

One thing that may help you cope at a time when nothing seems to be going right (the baby is crying even though you keep feeding him; your husband and other children are hungry; the children need washing, undressing, a bedtime story, a cuddle and being put to bed; and you're exhausted) is to remember that if you can possibly keep a sense of humour or at any rate a sense of proportion, it'll help. Try to untwist yourself if you're feeling strung up. Your ante-natal relaxation exercises may be useful, or you may find it unwinds you if you can do a ten-minute exercise routine or go for a run outside. Everyone feels like this sometimes and you just need to find your own way of coping with a time when all the demands are on you even though you may feel like being looked after as well!

Sometimes you may be able to link your baby's behaviour with something you have eaten earlier or the day before. Lots of babies get 'the wind' after their mothers have eaten cabbage. Others are uncomfortable after onions, unaccustomed Chinese food or alcohol. Trial and error will soon help you learn which foods you eat affect your baby in this way.

One final point. Changing your baby on to the bottle is highly unlikely to help. Bottle-fed babies are just as likely to suffer from evening crying as are breastfeds.

Q *What can I do about my baby's colic?* (See also preceding question.)
A Many cases of 'colic' are not due to intestinal spasm at all but simply due to hunger which causes periodic crying, often in the evening when the mother has little time to feed her baby and may be anxious about getting everything done for her baby, husband and other children. The answer here is to slow down and feed the baby as much as he wants, perhaps even on and off all evening for a few days. Recent research has shown that some cases of colic can be cured if the breastfeeding mother avoids all cows' milk and cows' milk products in her diet. An antispasmodic medicine is sometimes prescribed to treat colic but is by no means always successful. If your baby is so overwhelmed by your milk letting down in a rush that he swallows a lot of air trying to gulp the milk, this may give him tummy ache. Cope with this by collecting the initial fast flow and giving it to him by spoon afterwards. (See also page 174.)

Q *Can my baby's colic really be caused by cows' milk in my breast milk?*
A A study from Sweden suggested that this is likely. Twelve out

of nineteen colicky breastfed babies lost their colic when their mothers were put on a diet free from cows' milk protein. The colic reappeared on at least two further 'challenges' (in the form of a diet containing cows' milk for the mother). At four months, only four of the babies reacted with colic when their mothers had cows' milk in their diets, which fits in well with the observation that many babies tend to lose their colic after three or four months anyway. We know that whole molecules of cows' milk protein (and other dietary proteins) can be present in breast milk, and we know that colic is a well-recognised symptom of cows' milk protein intolerance, so the theory could well be right. As yet, though, it's unproven and it has been challenged by other researchers.

There is a suggestion that breastfed babies might benefit from exposure to 'foreign' proteins and other dietary substances in breast milk because it helps prepare their immunity system gradually for the switch to a mixed diet. However, certain babies, the colicky ones included, may be unable to cope with these food traces in breast milk and this inability to cope will be more likely if there is an allergic family history.

Some allergy experts suggest that the breastfeeding mother of a child with an allergic family history, or just with colic, should vary her diet so as to avoid a large intake of any one specified food, particularly cows' milk. Eggs, bananas, apples, oranges, strawberries, tomatoes, coffee and chocolate have also been associated with colic in the breastfed baby if the mother has too much of them.

Even a little of some foods in the mother's diet can cause an acute bout of colic lasting for a day in some babies. Beans, onions, garlic and rhubarb have each been observed to have this effect in some mother–baby pairs. Colic nearly always improves after the first three months. Weaning the baby on to cows' milk formula almost always makes colic worse and so is not advisable.

Q My friend says my milk doesn't look rich enough for my baby because it's bluish-white. What do you think?
A This is the normal colour of breast milk in many women, though you'll probably notice that the colour of your milk is different at the beginning and the end of a feed. This colour difference depends on its fat content. We're more used to the colour of cows' milk, but that doesn't make it a 'better' colour than breast

milk and certainly doesn't mean that it is in any way more suitable for babies.

When your colostrum changes into mature milk, you'll notice a change in consistency and colour from the thickish, yellowish colostrum to the thinner, bluish-white or creamy-white milk. Don't be alarmed by this and start thinking that your milk has suddenly lost its quality. The change is quite normal.

Q   My baby gets very excited when he's near me. Can he smell my milk?
A   Studies in France and England have found that a baby turns to a pad that has been placed next to his mother's breast in preference to a clean one which has no milk on it and has not been in contact with the breast. It is the breast contact that is most important because babies don't turn to pads soaked in their mother's expressed breast milk. Babies also prefer the smell of their own mother's breast to that of other mothers.

Just what it is on the mother's breast that produces this unique recognition is not known but it could be the smell of natural chemicals called pheromones which are hormone-like substances known to be vital in animal recognition systems.

Q   Is it true that vegans and vegetarians cannot produce good quality milk and so should not breastfeed their babies?
A   We really need to consider these two groups of people separately because their diets are very different from a breastfeeding point of view. Vegetarians usually eat some eggs, cheese, fish and foods other than vegetables, contrary to popular belief. Because of this their intake of vitamin B_{12} is usually adequate and does not need supplementing during everyday life, pregnancy or while breastfeeding. As far as we know, the breast milk of vegetarians is also perfectly healthy in other respects and interestingly contains high levels of polyunsaturated fatty acids. The implications of this are not clear. In many countries both vegetarian and vegan diets would be considered conventional.

Vegans eat no animal foods at all and are therefore at risk of being short of vitamin B_{12}, essential for the normal formation of red blood cells and the normal functioning of nervous tissue. Vegans must have enough vitamin B_{12} both during pregnancy and when breastfeeding and some experts think they should take supplements all the time. Studies have shown that when a vegan mother's diet is supplemented with this vitamin, her milk contains normal amounts of vitamin B_{12} and her baby is perfectly safe. Some vegetables and foods of vegetable origin contain vitamin B_{12} (yeast, soya beans, comfrey, wheatgerm and some fermented foods).

Q   Is it all right for me to breastfeed my friend's baby if he cries while he has been left with me?
A   There's no reason why you shouldn't, and it'll save her having to express milk to leave in a bottle for you to give him. Make sure you own baby gets enough, though! Wet nursing each other's babies is on the increase. One day we may even see a return of the old-fashioned and formerly widely accepted practice of wet nursing, with baby minders offering such a service.

While very young babies may be quite content to be breastfed by another woman, older ones sometimes object to the point of refusing to suck at all, especially if they are unfamiliar with the substitute mother. When we discuss the idea of wet nursing other people's babies, many women say they would feel quite happy to do so. Some say they often want to pick up someone else's crying baby to put him to the breast to comfort him. A few say that the mere thought of having a strange baby at their breast revolts them.

Q   My newborn baby doesn't ask for many feeds and isn't putting on enough weight. What should I do?
A   Your baby needs to be fed more often, so put him to the breast at least twice as frequently. The stimulus to your breasts from more frequent feeds will increase your milk supply over a few days, provided that your let-down is working well. Don't cut short the length of the feeds but let him suck for as long as he wants to. Some babies like to suck on and off for long periods, perhaps falling asleep every few minutes, and only start taking more 'formal' feeds when they are older and stronger.

Some babies need to be reminded that the breast is there before they ask for feeds and the smell of your skin and milk can help to do this. Other feeding stimuli are the sounds your body makes – your voice, heartbeats and tummy rumbles, the sight of you and the feel of you. A baby left lying alone in his cot has only the stimulus of his empty tummy to remind him of you and your breasts, and this isn't always enough, especially if he is of low birth weight, jaundiced, ill, or apathetic following the use of pethidine during your labour. Keep your uninterested baby with you as much as possible, either lying in your arms as you sit up, lying beside you as you sit or lie in bed, or in your arms or a sling as you do things. All the stimuli he'll receive from you will encourage him to ask for and to be alert enough to take the breast more often.

Q You give the impression that breastfeeding involves feeding the baby very frequently for months on end. Is this right?
A Babies are all different and some want more frequent feeding than others. During the early days, most mothers find that their babies settle better on frequent feeds. If your baby wants frequent feeds, you soon get used to it. Feeds become second nature and not big occasions to plan for. Sometimes they last a long time and other times only a few minutes. As they grow older, many babies ask for fewer feeds and some settle into their own individual 'routines' which may happen by chance to be roughly two-, three- or four-hourly feeds.

Sometimes you may find that your baby will want feeding much more often than usual. He may be extra hungry because he's growing fast, because he's ill, teething or just upset. If he needs more milk, your milk supply will catch up in two or three days if you let him feed as much as he wants. If not, just letting him have unrestricted access to your breast will soothe him.

Mothers who put their babies to the breast as often as the babies want to usually feed much more often than schedule feeders. Their feeds also seem more effortless because they are taken so much in their stride.

Q Are breastfed babies less likely to get nappy rash?
A One survey showed that bottle-fed babies are twice as likely to suffer from nappy rash as breastfed ones.

Q My baby has suddenly started fighting at the breast at three months. Can you help?
A It sounds as though your baby may be frustrated because you don't have enough milk. Three months is a common time for the supply to dwindle, usually because of insufficient stimulation of the

breasts by too few feeds. Try increasing your milk supply by feeding him much more often and for as long as he wants to suck. He should be happier within two or three days.

If your baby sleeps through the night, this may be jeopardising your supply as your breasts are unemptied for too long. Wake your baby to feed him or express some milk when you go to bed and if you wake up during the night with tense breasts. Waking the baby is much more efficient and quicker than expressing.

Q   I'm taking breast milk to the hospital each day for my baby who's in the special care baby unit, but I haven't a fridge. How should I store the milk?
A   Buy two ice packs (from a camping shop) and leave one at the hospital each day to be refrozen. At home, keep the bottle of milk with a frozen ice pack on top in a closed insulated container such as a freezer bag or a polystyrene picnic box, or even simply a cardboard box lined with newspaper. Keep the container in the coldest place you can find and use it for carrying the milk to the hospital too.

Q   Will I need special clothes when I'm breastfeeding?
A   The only clothes that are completely impractical are dresses that fasten at the back (because you can't undress or pull your dress up every time you want to feed your baby!). Blouses or dresses that do up in front are functional but you'll find they are very revealing when opened enough to feed your baby. Of course, this doesn't matter at all when you're at home alone or in front of people with whom you're not shy. It does matter, though, if you're with people who'd be embarrassed to see you half naked or with whom you feel shy. Sometimes it is possible to feed discreetly with a few lower buttons undone. The obvious answer is to wear clothes that can be pulled up just enough to let the baby feed but show nothing, such as jumpers, T-shirts, loose shirts or blouses with jumpers or tank tops over. Feeding a baby with your clothes pulled up just enough looks as though he is simply being cuddled, and this makes it much easier to feed in public.

Q   What about buying new bras for breastfeeding?
A   If you buy special nursing bras, choose them as late in your pregnancy as possible or, preferably, after your baby is born as they

may not fit properly otherwise. The type with one hook per cup is easiest to use, though you can also buy ones with a zip in each cup. Rows of tiny hooks and eyes make demand feeding difficult and are awkward to do up and undo discreetly in company. Many women wear ordinary bras to breastfeed and just pull the cup down to free the breast. This works well if the bra is not too built up, but it's sensible to make sure that the bra supports you well enough, is large enough and doesn't squash any part of the breast when pulled down, as this may lead to a blocked duct.

Q I have inverted nipples. Will I be able to breastfeed?
A Even though your nipples look inverted, they may not be truly inverted. Try pinching the skin above and below your nipple with your thumb and forefinger. If the nipple stands out, it isn't truly inverted and your baby will be able to suck easily. If your nipples stand out when you are sexually aroused, then you'll have no trouble breastfeeding. If the nipple never stands out by itself and can't be made to stand out, the hormonal changes of pregnancy will probably alter the tissues behind the nipple so as to allow it to stand out when the baby sucks. Some women wear breast shells inside their bra during pregnancy to encourage their nipples to stand out, but their value is unproven simply because the normal changes in pregnancy mentioned above make it difficult to know what has caused the improvement. If your nipples are truly inverted and pregnancy and breast shells have made no difference, your baby may still be able to suck easily if you 'make a biscuit' of your breast with your thumb and forefinger and offer it to him. Wearing breast shells for a few minutes before a feed may encourage the nipples to stand out, though you must latch your baby on quickly after removing a shell. Engorgement is the number one enemy of successful latching-on in women with inverted nipples, so avoid this at all costs.

Q What happens if my breasts are too big or too small – can I breastfeed?
A The size of the breasts is no indicator of success with breastfeeding. Women with small breasts are just as successful as women with large ones because the difference in size is due to

differences in the amount of fat and not necessarily of milk-producing tissue.

Q   Won't breastfeeding make my breasts sag?
A   Not if you wear a properly fitting, supporting bra that doesn't allow the heavier than usual breasts to sag and to stretch the elastic fibres in the skin and the fibrous connective tissue framework within the breasts. Once the skin is stretched, the breasts are likely to sag, especially when you stop breastfeeding and the milk-producing tissues shrink. For this reason, you might like to wear a bra at night. The other important thing to guard against is engorgement, as this stretches the skin. Changes in the shape of the breasts after having a baby are seen in bottle-feeders as well as breastfeeders and are due to having been pregnant, not to breastfeeding. Women who manage to keep their weight gain in pregnancy to a reasonable amount and who keep their weight stable afterwards will avoid stretching of the skin of the breasts due to being too fat.

Q   Don't you agree that breastfeeding is too animal-like and embarrassing to be acceptable in our society?
A   Embarrassment is the commonest reason given by mothers for choosing not to breastfeed. However, breastfeeding has so many advantages to both baby and mother that increasingly more mothers feel that bottle-feeding with cows' milk formula is unacceptable. Breastfeeding can and should be done quite discreetly in public, though if you have a baby that chokes, kicks in delight or makes obvious sucking noises, it isn't so easy. What we have to overcome is the feeling that breastfeeding mothers should be encouraged to stay inside their own homes to breastfeed, or in private rooms by themselves. Even some baby clinics shepherd mothers who want to breastfeed away from the public area, and breastfeeding mothers have been known to be turned out of public places like the town hall or the swimming bath even though they are feeding discreetly! Obviously it's no good to tell a mother that there's no need to be embarrassed because she very likely will be, especially if she's feeding for the first time or if she's naturally shy and retiring. Perhaps the best advice to be given is to say that as the breastfeeding mother knows she's doing the best thing for her baby, she should

allow this confidence in her actions to bolster her up in situations where other people make things embarrassing. Secondly, we should all have the courage of our convictions and explain to others that breastfeeding is normal, natural and best for the baby. Only by changing society's attitudes will breastfeeding become completely acceptable to everyone.

Q *Do I need to prepare my breasts or nipples for breastfeeding?*
A Rolling, rubbing and using creams have all been shown to be of no value at all and even breast shells for inverted nipples are of doubtful value. The only thing to remember is that soap washes away the natural secretions produced by the skin of the nipples and areolae. These secretions keep the nipples supple, provide natural waterproofing and also contain natural antiseptics, so you should avoid soap in the few weeks before your baby is due (in case the baby comes early), after the birth and while you are breastfeeding.

Q *When should I give my baby his first breastfeed?*
A As the sucking reflex is at its height soon after birth, put your baby to the breast within the first half hour. He may not want to suck straight away, so just hold him near the nipple and touch the corner of his mouth with your nipple from time to time. If you have had a Caesarean section, ask your husband or the nurse to help put your baby to the breast as soon as you come round from the general anaesthetic (or at once if you have had an epidural). Although the sucking reflex is at its height in the first half hour after birth, it certainly doesn't disappear after that. However, research has shown that a delay of eight hours or more after birth before the first feed reduces the chances of successful breastfeeding, and a delay of more than twelve hours increases the likelihood that the mother will stop breastfeeding in the first two weeks because of insufficient milk. With the right knowledge of how to breastfeed, even delays such as these make no difference to the success of breastfeeding. The sad fact is that hospitals that allow such delays (or encourage them) are likely to be those that encourage schedule feeding, discourage night feeds and put babies in the nursery at every opportunity. It is these factors that contribute most to breastfeeding failure.

Q   Can I breastfeed after a Caesarean section?
A   Yes. (See above question.) As your tummy will probably be tender, you'll need help to get your baby into a comfortable position for feeding. This may be with you lying on one side or with you sitting up and the baby propped up on pillows at your side, with his feet pointing the opposite way from the usual feeding position, and not across your tummy. Unrestricted breastfeeds are just as important for you as for any other mother in order to produce a good milk supply.

Q   My hospital has 'rooming-in'. What is this?
A   This simply means that each mother has her baby by her bed day and night and perhaps even in her bed at night. Rooming-in allows you to feed your baby on an unrestricted basis, which encourages the establishment of a satisfactory milk supply and also enables you to look at, talk to, hold and cuddle your baby as much as you like.

Q   Can I breastfeed my baby if he is premature?
A   If your baby is well enough to have milk feeds, he is certainly well enough to have your breast milk, though this may have to be given by tube (through his nose and down the gullet to the stomach).

The sucking reflex doesn't mature until a baby is between thirty-two and thirty-six weeks' gestation. If your baby is born early, the sucking reflex will mature at the equivalent time, so a baby born at twenty-nine, thirty or thirty-one weeks must be tube fed because he won't be mature enough to suck from you. However, from the equivalent of thirty-two weeks onwards, the breast can be offered from time to time, and he should show increasing interest once he has first sucked and tasted some milk. You might like to express a few drops first so that he can smell the milk on you. He may not be interested in sucking until he is the equivalent of thirty-six weeks, but the time spent trying before that will certainly not be wasted as it will give you the opportunity to hold him and get to know him. By regularly and frequently expressing (or pumping with an electric pump) your milk to be given to your baby by tube until he is able to suck from you, you will maintain your milk supply. *One thing to avoid is giving your breast milk to your baby in a bottle*, as it is much easier for him to suck from a bottle than from the breast and you might find it difficult or even impossible to interest him in the breast once he is used to the bottle.

Q Which is better for premature babies: breast milk or cows' milk formula?
A Many doctors believe that even very young (under thirty-two weeks) babies do better and are more healthy on breast milk though their growth rate may not be as fast as if they were given cows' milk formula. Babies of over thirty-two weeks (or the equivalent) thrive on breast milk.

It's fascinating that the breast milk of a mother whose baby was born pre-term is different in composition from full-term breast milk and more suitable for the particular needs of a relatively immature baby. This is why it is better for a mother to give her premature baby her own breast milk rather than for him to have breast milk from a milk bank, which will all have been donated from mothers producing milk suitable for full-term babies. Also, breast milk from a donor mother may have been heat treated to sterilise it before it is put in the milk bank. Sterilisation can destroy certain vitamins, antibodies and live cells and can alter the protein compositon of breast milk.

Q How do I express milk?
A Wash your hands and prepare a sterilised container for the milk if it is to be fed to the baby later. Make yourself comfortable. Hold the areola with your thumb above the nipple and your forefinger below and move your hand firmly backwards towards your chest. Now move your hand away, pressing your finger and thumb together and squeezing the milk along the ducts to the nipple. Carry on expressing once the milk is let down even though there are intervals between sprays. Move your hand from time to time to empty all the parts of the breast, and change to the other breast if the flow seems to be slowing. Change sides several times to collect enough milk for a whole feed so as to leave a feed for your baby if you are going out, you'll have to express after each feed for a couple of days in order to get enough. Leave the bottle in the fridge between times. Expressed milk should be deep frozen if it is to be kept for longer than two or three days.

Q I seem to leak an awful lot. Is there anything I can do about it?
A Frequent changes of absorbent non-stick paper or material pads inside your bra will help and a waterproof layer between the pad and your bra may help avoid embarrassing moments when milk soaks your dress. However, perhaps the best tip is to press firmly over the nipple with the ball of your thumb to stop the leaking.

Q Can I prevent myself getting mastitis or a breast abscess?
A These conditions can almost always be prevented following the breastfeeding techniques we have outlined. If you have a blocked duct, prompt treatment will prevent the stagnant milk from becoming infected and causing an abscess.

Q Can I stop my nipples getting sore when I breastfeed my baby?
A You can help prevent soreness by feeding your baby more often (perhaps the opposite of what you might have thought). Avoid using soap on your nipples and keep them dry between feeds by changing soggy breast pads and bras frequently. Expose your breasts to the air when you can: sunlight (or ultra-violet light from a lamp) clears up nipple soreness, and simply leaving your bra off under your clothes helps. Make sure your baby is latched-on comfortably and alter his feeding position from time to time. Prevent engorgement because the baby can't latch on properly to an overfull breast and will just chew on the nipple. If you still end up getting sore nipples, remember that the soreness rarely lasts for long and with perseverance feeds will soon be pain-free.

Q I'm sure I haven't enough milk for my baby. What should I do?
A You can increase your milk supply at any time simply by feeding your baby much more often and for longer at each feed, by night and day. Restricted feeding is the basic cause of insufficient milk, which in turn is the most common reason given by mothers who stop breastfeeding before they want to. Some mothers have insufficient milk because of an untrained let-down reflex, because their baby sucks poorly or because they themselves are eating too little and irregularly.

Q How often should I feed my baby and for how long at each feed?
A If your baby is thriving, feed him as often as he wants a feed. If

he is not gaining weight adequately, give him more feeds than he seems to need. Let him suck for as long as he want to, even if this is on and off for several hours from time to time. Most babies increase their mother's milk supply by demanding more feeds, but some babies (particularly small ones, those whose mothers had pethidine in labour, and babies with jaundice) become apathetic when they are hungry and can even starve themselves, apparently without protest. The more sucking time you allow your baby, the more milk you will have (provided he is sucking normally and so stimulating your breasts). Remember that an increase in sucking time takes about 36-48 hours to increase your milk supply.

Q When can I stop feeding my baby?
A Breastfeed your baby for a minimum of three to six months to give him the best start in life. Carry on feeding after that for as long as you like. More and more mothers are discovering the pleasure of feeding an older baby or young child and many allow their babies to decide when to stop breastfeeding. As long as you are enjoying the very special relationship a breastfeeding mother has with her older baby, baby-led weaning works very well.

Q I really think my husband is jealous of my baby breastfeeding, so wouldn't it be better for his sake to bottle-feed?
A Jealousy can be a problem for fathers and is partly caused by our society's emphasis on the breasts as sex objects rather than things to feed babies with. On a personal basis, explain to him the benefits of breast milk for your baby in the hopes that his unselfish desire to have the best for his baby will overcome his more selfish desire to have your breasts to himself. On a wider basis, do as much as you can (in your own family or even in schools if you can, by influencing teachers) to bring up boys knowing that breasts are primarily for babies, though they have an important sex function as well. There's no reason why you can't share your breasts with your husband and the baby.

Q Won't breastfeeding ruin my sex life?
A Some women feel more sexy during the months of breast-feeding and others less. They may feel different from one baby to another, or during any one lactation. Perhaps the worst killer of

sexual desire is tiredness, so if your baby wakes often at night, consider having the baby in bed with you and your husband simply so that you can feed him in bed without even having to wake up properly. There is no danger of smothering unless you or your husband go to bed drunk or drugged or unless either of you is extremely obese.

Q Can I restart my milk supply now my milk has dried up?
A Any woman can stimulate a supply of milk over a period of time by putting her baby to the breast regularly, by hand expressing or by pumping her breasts. Even if she hasn't had a baby, she can do this. Many women have breastfed adopted babies in this way and very many more have restarted their milk supply a few days, weeks, months or even years after stopping feeding.

Q Where can I get specialised help with breastfeeding?
A Mother-to-mother counselling is available from National Childbirth Trust breastfeeding counsellors and La Leche League leaders (addresses can be found on page 268). Increasingly more doctors and health visitors are interested and helpful, though some are still apt to suggest stopping breastfeeding or using complements of cows' milk formula at the drop of a hat.

Q Can I breastfeed my older baby if I get pregnant again?
A Yes, of course, though you should make sure you have an adequate, well-balanced diet to provide you, the unborn baby and the older baby with enough nutrients.

Q Does my baby need anything else to eat or drink while I'm breastfeeding?
A Not until three to six months at the earliest. Some mothers breastfeed completely for longer than this, though it's wise to introduce small amounts of food and drink from six months to accustom the baby to other tastes. Vitamins are unnecessary for the successfully breastfed baby *provided* the mother has a varied and nutritious diet. Research suggests, though, that dark-skinned babies in northern areas may be short of vitamin D because of the relative lack of sunlight (which manufactures vitamin D in the skin), so their mothers will be advised to give them vitamin D

supplements. Water and fruit juices are quite unnecessary before you start weaning. Fluoride supplements may be advisable if the level of fluoride in your water supply is low. Talk to your dentist about this.

Q I've heard that there is an aerosol spray containing chlorhexidine which helps prevent mastitis and nipple cracks. Is it worth getting one?
A No. There is no evidence from several studies that this spray prevents either nipple cracks or soreness, or that it is useful once you have got either. As for mastitis, such breastfeeding techniques as are outlined in this book are well known to be likely to prevent mastitis (with or without breast infection) anyway. Adjusting your technique will help cure mastitis, cracks and soreness if they do develop. An antibiotic is advisable for a true breast infection. Adequate precautions against cross-infection in hospital lower the risk of breast infection there.

Q My three-month-old totally breastfed baby is very fat. Should I start solids now and should I cut down his breastfeeds?
A There's no point in starting any other foods or drinks other than breast milk yet. Wait until he's six months old before you start giving him tastes of your family food of suitable consistency. Carry on breastfeeding him as and when he wants, for as long as he wants. The only problem fatness may cause at this age is soreness of the skin where chubby folds of skin rub together. If you keep his skin clean and dry, you can avoid this completely. You might like to reassure yourself that he's not spending too much time at the breast because this is the only way he can get your attention. Sometimes (but not always) more time spent talking to, playing with and showing things to a baby means less time with him at your breast, desperately trying to keep you with him.

Q My young baby is very healthy but seems to want to be fed almost all the time and I'm getting very frustrated because I can't get on with anything else. Is this normal?
A Your baby's behaviour is quite normal. Lots of babies go through stages lasting anything from a day or two to several weeks when they prefer to spend what seems like much of their waking

time at the breast. Sometimes this corresponds with a need to increase the milk supply, for example during a growth spurt, or after a cold or other illness when the milk supply may have fallen because of a decrease in the number of feeds. Check that you are not putting your baby down somewhere immediately after each feed. If you do, he will soon learn that the only way to stay close to you is to demand a breastfeed. Try using a sling to carry him in so that he is lulled by being next to you – you can go shopping, make beds, do housework and cook with it. It's only for a short part of his life that he'll be so very dependent on you. Whether you enjoy this time or hate it because of your frustration depends entirely on your attitude and, of course, attitudes can be changed. Experienced mothers and psychologists agree that babies who are given as much time as they want at the breast, and are cuddled or carried in their mother's arms, grow up to be *more independent* as toddlers than babies whose mothers' time and attention are rationed.

Carry out a time-and-motion analysis of your day and try to find ways of sitting or playing with your baby as much as you can. Mothers whose previous jobs were highly organised may find it difficult to do this and learn to relax and enjoy their new profession – motherhood – only with their second or third baby. Don't waste these early months of dependency with your first baby. Settle down, guilt-free, and run your new life as a proud mother, not as someone who sees a baby as an encumbrance and a hindrance to getting things done efficiently. So what if you never seem to finish what you're doing! Do it in several stages throughout the day instead, like hundreds of other mothers have learned to do. You'll probably find that it helps you relax if you make friends whom you can see from time to time. If you're alone with your baby a lot it's all too easy to worry.

Q   If I express milk from my breast, I can see drops of different coloured milk at the nipple. Some is creamy-white, some is thinner and bluish-white and some looks halfway between the two. Why is this?
A   This is because the composition of the milk changes according to whether it's expressed early or late in a feed (see page 34). Different milk reservoirs under the areola may be emptied at different rates, depending on the position in which the baby is feeding at the breast. Sometimes the milk in one reservoir may be

different in colour from that in other reservoirs because the gland it drains may not have been completely emptied at the previous feed. This means that at the same time you may see drops of bluish-white, thin, low-fat foremilk; thicker, creamy-white, high-fat hindmilk; and milk which is somewhere between the two owing to mixing of the milk in the ducts and reservoirs. Usually at the beginning of a feed most of the drops you see at the nipple are of foremilk, while towards the end most are of hindmilk. If the breast wasn't emptied completely during a feed, at the beginning of the next feed the drops you'll see will contain hindmilk (remaining in the reservoirs since the last feed), perhaps diluted slightly with some foremilk that has been pushed into the elastic-walled reservoirs since the last feed. Yet another reason for seeing drops of different colours is that some of the fifteen to twenty milk ducts from the milk glands may merge within the nipple (so there may be fewer openings at the nipple than there are glands, ducts and reservoirs). If one gland was emptied more thoroughly than another at the last feed and if their ducts merge in the nipple, then you may see milk halfway in colour between foremilk and hindmilk coming from that duct.

Q   My fully breastfed baby has eczema. What should I do?
A   Eczema is relatively much less common in babies who are fully breastfed and who have never received any cows' milk formula or any other food or drink. Although it is sometimes impossible to find a cause for eczema, it is certainly worth a try, especially if it is distressing for your baby.

First, make sure that nothing in contact with your baby's skin could be causing allergic contact eczema (dermatitis). Some babies are sensitive to wool, fabric softeners, detergent, various additives in washing powders, or the perfumes in disposable nappies, soap, talcum powder or cream. Check that you haven't mistaken dry skin for eczema. Dryness can be caused by too much washing with soap or by using a soap-free bath product.

Next, consider whether you are eating or drinking any particular food in excess. For example, are you drinking more than a pint of milk a day? That would represent a very large proportion of your total daily calorie intake in the form of one particular food. Certain foods may come through undigested in trace amounts in breast milk. If your baby is particularly susceptible (as may be the case if there is allergy on either side of the family) then trace amounts of one or more foods may be just enough to cause eczema or other allergic symptoms (such as colic, diarrhoea or a runny nose). Research work on this is still at an early stage, but it's certainly worth a trial of food exclusion because it won't hurt anyone and may just do the trick. Give up one food at a time (otherwise you won't know which one it was) for a week and watch what happens to your baby's skin. Start with cows' milk and other dairy products (remembering to replace the nutrients with other foods), then try giving up in turn eggs, wheat, corn, bananas, apples, oranges and other citrus fruits, strawberries, tomatoes, nuts, fish, shellfish, coffee and chocolate. Liaise with your paediatrician throughout if your child's eczema is severe. He will be delighted if you can find a cause.

Finally, if you become pregnant again, restrict your diet so that you never overindulge in any one particular food but instead eat a wide variety of foods. It's been shown that babies can be sensitised to foods their mothers eat even before they are born.

Q If my breastfed baby is allergic to something I have eaten how soon will he get a reaction?
A   There is no easy answer to this as the speed will depend on how quickly the food is absorbed into your bloodstream and hence into your milk, and on the type of allergic response. Some mothers notice allergic symptoms in their babies as soon as after the next breastfeed after the meal in question. Others report a delay of two to three days.

Q When will my baby start to sleep through the night?
A   No one can tell you because each baby is an individual and will start to sleep through the night only when he is ready. Babies wake at night for many reasons: they may be hungry (or thirsty); they may want to snuggle up to the breast for reassurance and comfort; they may be cold; or they may wake for no reason other than that their level of sleep has become light (as it does every so often during the night) and a noise, a light, a smell or some other stimulus has awoken them properly. A few breastfed babies sleep through the night after the first few weeks while others wake for many months or even years. Some babies wake several times, others once after the

parents have gone to bed. A few babies want to be at the breast more or less constantly during the night from time to time and the only way to cope with this is to have the baby in bed with you so that you can snooze.

Giving solids makes no difference to whether or not a baby sleeps through the night. Bottle-fed babies do sleep more than breastfed ones and also tend to sleep through the night sooner, but this doesn't mean to say that you should put a night-waker on to cows' milk formula. The advantages of breast milk to the baby are far too important to be thrown away that lightly.

Advice often given to parents of a baby who wakes at night is to let him cry in his cot every night for three nights, by when he'll have realised that he might just as well not bother. It's impossible to find out scientifically exactly what psychological harm this sort of treatment might do but it certainly seems to go against all natural human responses. Research has shown however that babies who are left to cry a lot cry more as one-year-olds. Parents who are uninfluenced by current advice on baby care (which is all based on as much separation from them as possible) will take the baby into bed with them, so that he is no trouble to feed when he wakes. It would be a tremendous help to parents-to-be if ante-natal preparation classes stressed the fact that *night waking is normal*. This might help prevent the resentment felt by parents who think they have an abnormal or even 'naughty' baby if he happens to do what the vast majority of babies do – wake at night. Patterns of sleep vary enormously even in any one baby. Your baby may wake several times most nights but occasionally have a long stretch of sleep. If he is usually a heavy sleeper, he may have a wakeful night from time to time, perhaps if you have eaten something that disagrees with him.

If you drink a lot of caffeine-containing drinks, or if you smoke, it might help your baby to sleep longer if you cut both these habits out or at least down.

Q When my baby wakes me at night I feel so annoyed at having my sleep broken that I can't go back to sleep. How can I make him sleep?
A You can't make him, unless your doctor were to prescribe strong, potentially addictive hypnotics or sedatives that might have other undesirable side effects as well. You can encourage him to wake less by keeping him with you during the day. This way he'll

probably sleep slightly less in the day and more at night. Hopefully he'll eventually become more in tune with your own patterns of sleeping, waking and feeding.

Your attitude to his night-waking is all-important because your annoyance may colour your whole feeling towards him. Try to accept that his behaviour is normal. Try going to bed earlier yourself, so that you get more hours resting in bed, or have some naps during the day. If you rest or sleep by your baby during the day every time he sleeps, then your sleep deficit will be reduced. Concentrate on the positive aspects of night-waking, if you can, instead of the negative ones. When your baby wakes you, cuddle him as he feeds and enjoy the feel of his warm, soft body nestling against you. If you feed him lying down in bed with the light off, you'll probably both go back to sleep sooner than if you sit with the light on and wind and change him afterwards. Put a thick nappy on at the beginning of the night so he probably will manage without a change at all. If he seems to be windy, just sit him up for a minute or two.

Q   *What is the normal number of night feeds for a breastfed baby?*
A   There is no one 'normal' number. It is just as normal for a baby to suck at the breast on and off for much of the night with short naps every now and then as it is for him to sleep right through from the age of a few weeks. What your baby does will depend on his age and individual sleep pattern. Very young babies tend to wake at night more often than older ones. Some babies learn to follow their mothers' patterns of wakefulness and sleep, especially if they are close to their mothers all day and night, while others have their own. The most unhelpful thing you can do, though we all do it with our first babies, is to compare your baby's sleeping habits with those of another baby. You'll be doing yourself a favour if you simply accept whatever your baby does. If waking at night makes you tired, sleep or rest during the day whenever your baby falls asleep. It's very easy to get stuck in the rut of believing that your body needs a certain amount of sleep. In fact most people can get by with less sleep than they usually have with no ill effects. Many non-western societies never normally have one long period of sleep as we tend to do.

When you're in hospital you may be encouraged to note down the time of each breastfeed. This is for the benefit of the nursing and medical staff who want to check that your baby is getting enough feeds. When you get home, try not to look at the clock at night. It's far less disconcerting if you snooze through a feed rather than watch the minutes ticking by.

Q My eight-month-old breastfed baby screams if I leave him with anyone else. Is this abnormal?
A It's part of the normal course of development for a baby to become attached to his mother, provided he is given enough chance to do so. It's been said by one expert that if a child of between six months and two years old *doesn't* get upset when his mother leaves him, he's showing abnormal behaviour.

Q Can I breastfeed my baby after having plastic surgery on my breasts to make them smaller (a reduction mammoplasty)?
A Yes you can. However, whether or not you manage to breastfeed your baby fully will depend on the type of operation you had, how much glandular tissue was removed, how many milk ducts were cut and whether the cut ends of the ducts have managed to join up with patent ducts so that the milk can get from the glands to the nipple. If you have had this sort of operation, the only way to know whether breastfeeding will be successful is to try it and see. Even if you only manage to give your baby some milk each day, it will be worth it for him and for you. If you are contemplating having such an operation before you have children, tell your surgeon that one day you will want to breastfeed your babies.

Q I started using a nipple shield because my nipples were sore. The soreness is now gone but my baby isn't interested in sucking unless the shield is there.
A One of the several disadvantages of a nipple shield is that some babies get so used to it that they won't take the breast at all without one. You'll have to be rather clever if you want to stop using it. Try cutting a little piece of the rubber away after each feed, so the baby gradually gets used to the feel and taste of your skin again. Or, once you baby is sucking well with the shield in place, you may be able to slip it out without him noticing.

You're wise to be concerned about using a shield because your milk supply may fall if you use it for long. The stimulation of the nerve endings in the skin of the nipple and areola is bound to be less with a shield in place, so your pituitary gland's prolactin and oxytocin output will fall.

What's more, a nipple shield may harbour bacteria or thrush unless it's really well cleaned after use. Unless you absolutely have to, avoid using one at all.

Q Do some mothers have more milk than others?
A Undoubtedly, yes. However, each woman can increase her milk supply to its own individual full potential and there's every reason to suppose that almost every healthy and well-nourished woman is capable of feeding her baby adequately if she knows what to do and wants to do it. Perhaps underlying this question is the observation that on a four-hourly schedule of breastfeeding (still wrongly recommended by some authorities) a few women produce plenty of milk. These are the women who undermine the confidence of the majority who need more feeding sessions than this to stimulate their milk supply sufficiently. The answer is not to take any notice of how much milk anyone else has but simply to do what you and your baby need to do in order for him to be happy and well nourished.

Q My baby didn't want many feeds on the first day after he was born though I was quite ready to give him the breast whenever he wanted. Why was this?
A Provided he wasn't jaundiced, pre-term, ill or drugged because of drugs you were given before or during labour, then it's most likely that he was just proving to you that the protein level of colostrum is much higher than that of mature milk. The higher protein level of colostrum enables newborn babies to go longer between feeds, which may be nature's way of ensuring that the newly delivered mother has a chance to get some sleep too.

Q I give ante-natal classes and I'm concerned that if I tell mothers that breast milk is best for their babies then the mothers who decide not to breastfeed, or can't breastfeed, will feel guilty about bottle-feeding. Is it reasonable to make them feel like this?
A You should respect the right of every mother to make an *informed* decision about how her baby is to be fed. If she isn't told

the truth about the benefits of breastfeeding, then she can't make an informed decision. If she decides not to breastfeed even though she's got all the facts at her fingertips, that's up to her. The argument about the guilt (or disappointment) of the mother who *can't* breastfeed is another matter. First, the vast majority of women who 'fail' to breastfeed for as long as they want to could in fact succeed if they were given the right help and advice. Only a tiny number of women will actually be unable to breastfeed at all (see page 146). Virtually every woman can give her baby some breast milk, even if he also has cows' milk or other formula, and it should be stressed ante-natally that even a little breast milk is better than none at all, though, of course, complete breastfeeding is the best of all.

Really the argument is a non-starter. The good you'll be doing by encouraging more mothers to breastfeed far outweighs any bad you'll do by possibly making a few mothers who choose to bottle-feed feel guilty. It wouldn't be a bad idea to discuss with your group the fact that it's not only the baby who misses out if he's bottle fed. The mother will miss out on lots of things too! (See page 36.)

Q   Do I need to take extra vitamin D if I'm breastfeeding?
A   We now know that sunshine is a far better source of vitamin D than any food. Vitamin D produced in the skin after exposure to sunlight can be stored and used during the winter months. It makes sense for the woman who is pregnant or breastfeeding to get as much sun as she can and for babies to be allowed to sunbathe when possible, taking care to avoid over-exposure (see also page 29).

Although sunshine is the most important source of vitamin D it's sensible to ensure that your diet during pregnancy and breast-feeding includes plenty of vitamin D-containing foods (margarine, fatty fish, eggs and butter). For mothers who have little exposure to sunlight or whose diet is deficient in this vitamin, vitamin D supplements are available.

Q   My nipple is bleeding. Is this because it is slightly cracked?
A   A crack in the nipple is the commonest cause of bleeding. Do everything you can to heal the crack and prevent it happening again. There is no need to stop the baby from feeding because the blood will not hurt him.

If there is no crack, then bleeding seen at the nipple can be caused by a variety of conditions including a benign (non-malignant) tumour called an intraduct papilloma. This bleeding will almost certainly stop once breastfeeding is established.

There are other rarer causes of bleeding including other tumours and this is why, unless you are sure that the blood is coming from a crack, it is wise to consult your doctor.

Q *If my baby is ill, is it better for him to be bottle-fed?*
A Certainly not. Your sick baby should have the best nutrition available. This is also the time when he needs the comfort of being at his mother's breast as usual. It's interesting that if your baby has an acute respiratory illness with difficulty in breathing, breastfeeding is easier for him to cope with. The bottle-fed baby tends to breathe in a more gasping fashion between swallows.

Q *My eight-month-old baby wants such frequent feeds that it's beginning to annoy me. I lead an active life and my friends disapprove of my feeding him so often. How can I stop him feeding so often?*
A How often a baby wants to feed depends on his personality, how hungry and thirsty he is, how tired he is and on whether or not he is well and happy. In other words, there may be some specific reason why your baby sometimes or always wants frequent feeds or he may just be asking for what is perfectly normal and desirable for him.

It's worth considering whether your active life is conflicting with your baby's best interests. We're not suggesting that you should necessarily cut down on what you do, but perhaps you might give your baby more of your time and attention, rather than spend it so freely on activities and other people. Your baby is your prime responsibility at present. The investment of time and love that you put into him now will pay off massively over the years. It's all too easy for a sociable person to sit with her baby on her lap and to talk to her friends constantly. The baby's only way of getting any attention is to ask for a feed, when all he might (quite justifiably) want is for her sometimes to talk to and play with him. Try chatting up your baby as well as your friends. You may find that he doesn't need to spend so much time at the breast then. Even if he does, he'll benefit from having you pay attention to him.

Q My baby has a cleft lip. Surely bottle-feeding will be easier?
A No. In fact breastfeeding may be easier because the soft breast can be moulded round the cleft in the lip and so provide a seal, unlike the rubber of a bottle teat, so that the nipple and areola can be held in the baby's mouth by suction. It's most important for you to ensure that your breasts don't become too full, which would make it difficult for your baby to get a seal with his lips. Express some milk if necessary before a feed and feed frequently to avoid engorgement.

Appendix

Recommended reading list

When reading anything written with the aim of helping you feed, bring up or look after your child, remember that the information is there for you to sift and use if it seems right for you and your family. No author can get everything right and certainly no author can address himself to each individual reader. It's up to you to read what seems most suitable, discuss it with friends, family, professional advisers and counsellors, and then to act on a mixture of this information plus a good helping of common sense.

The following books and articles on breastfeeding, mothering, childbirth, bonding and sleeping will be of interest to anyone who has enjoyed *Breast is Best*.

The Womanly Art of Breastfeeding, La Leche League International, (new edition 1981)

The Experience of Breastfeeding, Sheila Kitzinger, Pelican Books

Breastfeeding, the Biological Option, G. J. Ebrahim, The Macmillan Press

The Tender Gift: Breastfeeding, Dana Raphael, Schocken Books, New York

Mothering your Nursing Toddler, Norma Jane Bumgarner, PO Box 5064, Norman, Ok. 73070, USA

The Breastfeeding Book, Máire Davies, Century Publishing

The Breast Book, Drs Penny and Andrew Stanway, Granada Publishing

Breast-Feeding and Natural Child Spacing, Sheila Kippley, Penguin Books

Abreast of the Times, R. M. Applebaum MD, 7914 SW 104th St, Miami, Fla. 33156, USA

'Breastfeeding and Drugs in Human Milk', Gregory J. White, MD and Mary Kerwin White, *Veterinary and Human Toxicology*, Vol. 22, supplement 1, 1980, available from La Leche League

Breastfeeding: A Guide for the Medical Profession, Ruth A. Lawrence, The C.V. Mosby Company

Human Milk in the Modern World, Derrick B. and E. F. Patrice Jelliffe, Oxford University Press

Women as Mothers, Sheila Kitzinger, Fontana Books

Distress and Comfort, Judy Dunn, Fontana/Open Books

The Continuum Concept, Jean Liedloff, Futura Publications

Mothering, Rudolph Schaffer, Fontana/Open Books

Breastfeeding and the Mother, Ciba Foundation Symposium 45 (new series), 1976, Elsevier, Excerpta Medica, New York

The Psychology of Childbirth, Aidan Macfarlane, Fontana/Open Books

Pregnancy and Childbirth, Sheila Kitzinger, Michael Joseph

Maternal–Infant Bonding, Marshall H. Klaus and John H. Kennell, The C.V. Mosby Company

New Life, Arthur and Janet Balaskas, Sidgwick and Jackson

The Family Bed, Tine Thevenin, PO Box 16004, Minneapolis, Mn. 55416, USA

The Pears Encyclopaedia of Child Health, Drs Andrew and Penny Stanway, Pelham Books

The Baby and Child Book, Drs Andrew and Penny Stanway, Pan Books

Breast pumps

These are necessary only in certain situations (see below) and most breastfeeding mothers will never need to use one. However good a pump is, it is never as effective either at milking the breast or at stimulating the milk supply as is a healthy baby. Electric pumps are more efficient than hand pumps or hand expression of the breast. If it seems likely that breastfeeding will be impossible for some weeks, for example with a very small pre-term baby, then electric pumping is the best method of milking the breast as it is the least tiring for the mother. Her hands can become very tired with prolonged hand pumping.

Before use, all parts of a pump in contact with the milk should be sterilised, especially if the milk is to be given to a baby. Position the flange (the funnel-shaped receiving end of the pump) so that the nipple rests at the inside of the upper part. This means that, during pumping, the nipple is drawn in and out and the contact with the side of the flange encourages the let-down of the milk. Spread the first few drops of milk over the skin in contact with it, so that the flange can slide over the skin easily. Don't press the flange too tightly against your breast as this could obstruct the milk ducts or reservoirs. It's sensible to try to start the let-down of the milk before the pump is used by massaging the breast and by hand expression. Massage of the breast during pumping will help the flow of milk and encourage further let-downs. The pump should be changed to the other breast when the milk flow diminishes or stops. You can change from one breast to another several times during a pumping session, just as you would with a baby at your breast. At first, only very small amounts of milk (such as a quarter of an ounce) may be collected.

Because pumping is not as good as a baby at stimulating the milk supply the pump should be used *at least as often* as babies generally want a feed. Four-hourly is rarely enough and *a minimum* of eight to ten sessions (two- to three-hourly) should be aimed at. The milk supply can usually be increased by increasing the number and length of pumping sessions.

When you might need a breast pump

1 When your baby is too immature or too ill to get milk from the breast himself.

2 In the rare event that you are taking essential drugs which would be harmful to your breastfed baby via your milk. Your pumped milk will be thrown away but your milk supply can be kept going until you are off the drugs and the baby can be put to the breast again.

3 In the rare event that you have a serious infection which temporarily precludes your baby from being with you and having your milk. Your pumped milk will be thrown away but your milk supply can be kept going until your infection is under control (usually very soon) and your baby can be put to the breast again.

4 If your baby has to stay in hospital and you are unable to stay with him (or vice versa). You can pump your milk, store it under suitable conditions and take it into the hospital when you go.

5 If you are building up a supply of milk before taking delivery of an adopted baby.

6 If you are building up your milk supply again after weaning too early.

7 If you want to collect milk to leave for your baby if you have to go out without him.

8 If you work away from home and want to collect milk for him at work or just keep your milk supply going by regular pumping at work.

9 If you have truly inverted nipples, when a pump might be useful to bring out the nipple as far as possible just before a feed. *Immediately* after using the pump for a minute or so, put your baby to the breast.

Breast pumps are often used unnecessarily, especially in hospitals, because they are there, because man-made intervention in nature's process is so attractive to those who don't fully understand the way breastfeeding works, and because many mothers have learnt a poor breastfeeding technique. *If it's possible for your baby to breastfeed, it's far better for him and for you, so only pump if essential.* Frequently a baby is given cows' milk formula complements from a bottle, refuses to suck at the breast (because he has quickly learnt to bottle-suck) then, because his mother is determined to breastfeed, she pumps her milk and gives it by bottle. To avoid this it's best not to give the baby a bottle in the first place! Only rarely is it necessary to stop breastfeeding temporarily because of nipple soreness or cracking but, if you have to, it's less painful to hand-express your milk than to use a pump.

Types of breast pump

NB Prices were correct at time of going to press. The prices of the various electric pumps reflect to some extent their sturdiness and the quality of their engineering. In general, the larger the electric pump, the quicker the suction is built up, which means that for some mothers, pumping is quicker overall.

● *The Egnell Breast Pump* (electric). A Swiss pump distributed in the UK by Eschmann Bros and Walsh Ltd, Peter Road, Lancing,

Sussex (tel. 0903 761122). It is available also from medical supply houses and on hire from the National Childbirth Trust's pump agents (tel. 01 221 3833 for details). This pump is quiet, efficient, has variable suction with a resting phase and a slight positive pressure phase, and has two sizes of funnel (for different shaped breasts). It works by the suction applied to the breast together with the stimulation of the nipple and areola against the side of the flange. It weighs 11 kg and costs £596 plus VAT.

● *The Whittlestone Physiological Breast Milker* (electric). This is available from Y. Procuta, PO Box 17, Cambridge, New Zealand. This pump is more expensive than the Egnell pump but has a natural action as the soft foam lining of the breast cups milks the breasts by gentle, rhythmical compression aided by adjustable suction. It also saves time as both breasts can be milked at once. It is comfortable to use.

● *The Axicare Breast Pumps* (electric). A range of four pumps of varying size and price developed by Colgate Medical Ltd, 1 Fairacres Estate, Dedworth Road, Windsor, Berkshire SL4 4LE (tel. 07535 60378).

The CM10 is an automatic pump with an automatic sucking rhythm and variable suction strength. A carrying case is an optional extra. It weighs 5.5 kg and costs £258 plus VAT.

The CM8 is a semi-automatic pump which provides a constant vacuum, the strength and duration of which are controlled by the mother to suit herself, using the tip of a finger. A carrying case is an optional extra. It weighs 2 kg and costs £148 plus VAT.

The CM6 is a smaller version of the CM8. It comes with a carrying case, weighs 1.3 kg and costs £135 plus VAT.

The CM4 (Mini Breast Pump) is an even smaller (4″×3″×2″) semi-automatic pump which weighs 0.8 kg and costs £53 plus VAT.

● *The Medela Pump* (electric). Swiss pump similar to the Egnell and distributed by Vickers Medical, Priestly Road, Basingstoke, Herts (tel. 0256 29141). It is available on hire from La Leche League and costs £510 plus VAT.

Electric pumps are available for hire or on loan from some hospital maternity and special care baby units, and for sale from medical supply houses and some chemists. The Axicare CM6 pump is available on hire from Natural Joy, 1 Howard Close, London N11 (tel. 01 368 1077). This company also sells the Mini Breast Pump.

● *Hand pumps*
The Kaneson Pump, a Japanese pump distributed by Kimal Scientific Products Ltd, Unit E, Eskdale Road, Industrial Estate, Uxbridge, Middlesex (tel. 0895 59419), is a syringe-action pump that can be converted into a feeding bottle. It costs £7.00 including postage and packing and VAT. This pump is also available from some National Childbirth Trust pump agents (tel. 01 221 3833 for details).

Similar pumps to the Kaneson are the ones distributed by Colgate Medical – the *Axipump*, (£5.25) – and the *Robbins Nurser* (£6.58), available from some chemists or direct from the distributors: Robbins Medical Supplies Ltd, Dept RN, Otterburn, 22 The Avenue, Hitchin, Herts (tel. 0462 4899). They will send the pump by express mail at an extra charge.

These and other hand pumps of varying efficiency are available from chemists' shops, many by order only, which can take a long time. The cheapest and simplest pumps consist of a plastic or glass collecting chamber with a rubber bulb to produce the suction. Examples of these are the Saffron Breast Reliever and the Suba Seal. Milk collected using such pumps is likely to contain large amounts of bacteria because the rubber bulbs inevitably get some milk inside and are difficult to clean. Bacteria thrive on the milk residue and contaminate the next collection of milk. The pumps are also not very effective at removing milk from the breast.

Other useful information

The Lact-Aid Nursing Supplementer
Available from Resources in Human Nurturing International, Box 6861, Denver, Co. 80206, USA and from La Leche League and the National Childbirth Trust. A useful information booklet comes with the Lact-Aid. Further information about how to use the Lact-Aid if you want to breast-feed an adopted baby or simply get your milk supply back is also available from the above address. A Lact-Aid is also useful to teach a bottle-fed baby to suck properly at the breast.

Colgate Medical Ltd is working on a supplementer similar to the Lact-Aid but using a plastic bottle instead of a plastic bag. While much cheaper (£5) than the Lact-Aid, initial criticisms include not being able to disguise the bottle under clothing so as to feed discreetly, and that the tube is too stiff and thick for the baby to accept along with the nipple. Hopefully the latter problem will be ironed out easily.

The National Childbirth Trust
9 Queensborough Terrace, Bayswater, London W2 3TB (tel. 01 221 3833). The Breastfeeding Promotion Group has a wide range of information on breastfeeding including leaflets and recommended books. The NCT also sells its own brand of nursing bra.

La Leche League of Great Britain
BM3424, London WC1V 6XX (tel. 01 404 5011). Besides its useful manual, *The Womanly Art of Breastfeeding*, La Leche League also provides a good deal of other information, including:

● *For the blind or visually handicapped*. Many publications in Braille, on cassette tape or reel-to-reel. Ask for LLLI's special publications list – *BRL*.

● *Information sheets and reprints*. Over 200 of these are available on many aspects of breastfeeding and child care. A price list will be sent on request. Please enclose a stamped self-addressed business-size envelope. For information in languages other than English, ask for the translation list (No. 508).

Index

Non-fiction

☐	**The Money Book**	Margaret Allen	£4.95p
☐	**Fall of Fortresses**	Elmer Bendiner	£1.75p
☐	**The Love You Make**	Peter Brown and Steven Gaines	£2.95p
☐	**100 Great British Weekends**	John Carter	£2.95p
☐	**Last Waltz in Vienna**	George Clare	£1.95p
☐	**Walker's Britain**	Andrew Duncan	£5.95p
☐	**Travellers' Britain**	Arthur Eperon	£2.95p
☐	**The Tropical Traveller**	John Hatt	£2.95p
☐	**The Lord God Made Them All**	James Herriot	£2.50p
☐	**The Neck of the Giraffe**	Francis Hitching	£2.50p
☐	**A Small Town is a World**	David Kossoff	£1.00p
☐	**Prayers and Graces**	Allen Laing illus. by Mervyn Peake	£1.25p
☐	**Best of Shrdlu**	Denys Parsons	£1.50p
☐	**The New Small Garden**	C. E. Lucas Phillips	£2.50p
☐	**Thy Neighbour's Wife**	Gay Talese	£2.50p
☐	**Dead Funny**	Fritz Spiegl	£1.50p
☐	**Future Shock**	Alvin Toffler	£2.95p
☐	**The World Atlas of Treasure**	Derek Wilson	£6.50p

All these books are available at your local bookshop or newsagent, or can be ordered direct from the publisher. Indicate the number of copies required and fill in the form below

12

....

Name_____
(Block letters please)

Address_____

_____

Send to CS Department, Pan Books Ltd, PO Box 40, Basingstoke, Hants
Please enclose remittance to the value of the cover price plus:
35p for the first book plus 15p per copy for each additional book ordered
to a maximum charge of £1.25 to cover postage and packing
Applicable only in the UK

While every effort is made to keep prices low, it is sometimes
necessary to increase prices at short notice. Pan Books reserve
the right to show on covers and charge new retail prices which
may differ from those advertised in the text or elsewhere